THE GREATEST GENERATION *of* ORTHOPEDISTS

The visionaries, pioneers, healers, organizers and doers who built the modern practice of orthopedic and spine care -- and have since passed on.

by

ROBIN YOUNG
Publisher and Editor

TRACEY ROMERO, ELIZABETH HOFHEINZ
AND WALTER EISNER
Contributing Writers

THE GREATEST GENERATION OF ORTHOPEDISTS

Copyright © 2023 by RRY Publications LLC

All Rights Reserved.
For information about permission to reproduce selections from this book, write to Permissions, RRY Publications LLC.

For information about special discounts for bulk purchases, please contact RRY Publications LLC at www.ryortho.com.

Book design and jacket cover: Dana Lertch

FIRST EDITION

ISBN: 978-0-9779648-4-0

This book is dedicated to Biloine Whiting Young, a prolific writer, traveler, historian and my first and best editor.

It is also dedicated to the magnificent men and women who set up orthopedic and spine practices in the small towns and big cities all over North America between 1960 and 1990.

One patient at a time, these pioneers, visionaries, doers and healers, changed lives in profound ways and quite incidentally, created the largest sector of medicine.

CONTENTS

Introduction	*11*
Architects of Modern Orthopedic and Spine Surgery	15
Champ Leroy Baker Jr.	19
Lew Bennett	21
Adele Ludin Boskey	24
Antonio (Tony) Castellvi	27
John S. Collis Jr.	29
D. Kay Clawson	32
Lawrence Douglas Dorr	35
William F. Enneking	39
Albert B Ferguson Jr.	41
Freddie Fu	43
John Samuel Gould	47
Frank Gunston	49
Harry N. Herkowitz	51
David S. Hungerford	53
Frank Jobe	56
Norman A. Johanson	59
Kiyoshi Kaneda	61
Michael A. Kelly	64

Max E. Link	66
John Thomas Makley	68
Thomas Mallory	70
Henry J. Mankin	73
Bruno Melzi	75
Dane A. Miller	78
Maurice Edmond Muller	82
Arthur M. Pappas	86
Charles Ray	88
Charles A. Rockwood Jr.	91
Christoph Röder	93
Leon Root	95
Richard Rothman	97
Mitchell Seyedin	100
Russell E. Windsor	102
Willem Zeegers	104

Regional Founders, Pioneers and Champions of Modern Orthopedic and Spine Surgery	107
Albert Bernard Accettola	109
Dan Adair	110
Frank J. Boutin Sr.	112
David Lance Bowles	114
Glenn Blish Carpenter	115
Robert C. Coddington	116
Frank F. Cook	118
Eugene "Gene" R. Corasanti	120
David C. Cottrell II	122
John E. Davis	124
Leo De Souza	125
Jeffrey Thomas DeHaan	127

Robert Leonard Diaz	128
William "Lonnie" Dillon	129
John Elliot	131
Clint Devin	133
Leonard D. Emond	135
Timothy M. George	136
Walter T. Gilsdorf	139
Pau Golano	140
Todd Graham	142
Frank Benton Gray	144
Eugene "Gene" Frank Gulish	146
Armen Charles Haig	148
William H.B. Howard	149
Joseph A. Izzi Sr.	151
Jesse George Jackson	152
Walter "Bill" Hughey King Jr.	154
Petar Kokan	155
Alfred Kritter	156
Seung "Sam" Chan Lee	157
Dean Lorich	158
Bernard Allan Lublin	160
Dean Maar	161
Theodore Maravich	163
Anthony F. Merlino	164
Gary Wayne Miller Sr.	166
James E. Mraz	167
Marvin E. Mumme Jr.	168
Stephen Minick Neely	170
Cecil H. Neville Jr.	171
Stanford M. Noel	172
Donald Paarlberg	174

Mark Palumbo	175
Victor Panitch	177
John P. Park	179
Preston Philips	180
Thomas Lemuel Presson	182
Gurdev Purewal	184
Mario Randelli	186
John F. Raycroft	188
Robert Ernest Ribbe	190
Sheldon Roger	192
Raymond Donald Santucci	193
Francis (Frank) Henry Schildgen	195
R.J. Black Schultz	196
Sidney Schultz	197
Richard E. Senghas	198
John "Jack" Haines Shertzer	200
William H. Simon	202
Manmohan Singh	204
Robert Small	205
Otto K. Stewart	206
Elton Strauss	207
Howard Sturtz	208
Steven W. Theis	209
Michael Steven Thompson	210
Craig Tifford	212
Ralph Ilian Touma	214
Thomas Frank Trainer	215
James Edwin White	216
Richard P. Whittaker	218
Robert Michael Yanchus	220
Epilogue	*223*

INTRODUCTION

The years between 1970 and 2000 are, arguably, the golden years of orthopedics and spine surgery.

It was during this period that the great leaps in hip, knee, spine and extremity patient outcomes occurred.

It is also during this period that approximately 200,000 orthopedic and spine surgeons were trained in their craft and calling.

Jeffrey Thomas DeHaan, for example, brought orthopedic surgery to Texarkana, Texas and served that community for 36 years.

Or, Howard Sturtz, one of the pioneers of arthroscopic surgery, treated tens of thousands of patients in San Francisco.

Victor Panitch, Chief of Staff at two hospitals, brought orthopedics to central Massachusetts. Ralph Gessner, in practice for 45 years, brought orthopedics to New Orleans.

Norman Johanson, Professor at the Lewis Katz School of Medicine and Chief of Orthopedics at Hahnemann University until it closed in 2019. Thirty seven years serving patients.

Of this generation, about half (based on records we've compiled) served in the military – most in the Vietnam War.

These were the first surgeons trained in large joint arthroplasty, spine fusion, shoulder and extremity surgery and built the largest practice in medicine, serving more patients each year than any other.

This generation is also distinguished for its volunteer work.

Robert Ernest Ribbe of Grand Rapids Michigan, for example, was a member of the Christian Medical/Dental Society through which he volunteered to treat patients at no charge in Kenya, Romania, and Taiwan. He also spent almost 20 years ministering to prisoners.

Richard Senghas, M.D., former member of the Editorial Board for the Journal of Bone & Joint Surgery, brought the practice of orthopedic surgery to Worcester, Massachusetts. He would eventually serve as President of the medical staff at Framingham Union Hospital and clinical instructor at the University of Massachusetts Medical School in Worcester.

After more than 30 years treating orthopedic patients, Dr. Senghas 'retired' and entered Pope St. John XXIII National Seminary, served as chaplain intern at Wellesley College and Central Main Medical Center and at age 70, in 1998, was ordained Catholic priest for the Diocese of Maine.

There are thousands more examples.

In 2022: Dr. Senghas died at age 94. Dr. Ribbe died at age 83. Dr. Johansen died at age 72. Dr. DeHaan died at age 66, De. Sturtz died at age 87 and Dr. Panitch died at age 90.

The first generation of orthopedic and spine surgeons is passing.

This book celebrates the architects of modern orthopedics and spine as well as the visionaries, champions and regional leaders.

These men and women are the Greatest Generation of orthopedists ever.

They were the visionaries, pioneers, healers, organizers and doers who built modern orthopedic and spine care.

Finally, I hope the individual stories of this Greatest Generation, paint the truest picture of how this consequential and global medical practice came to be.

Robin Young – January 2023

Architects *of* Modern Orthopedic *and* Spine Surgery

George W. Bagby II

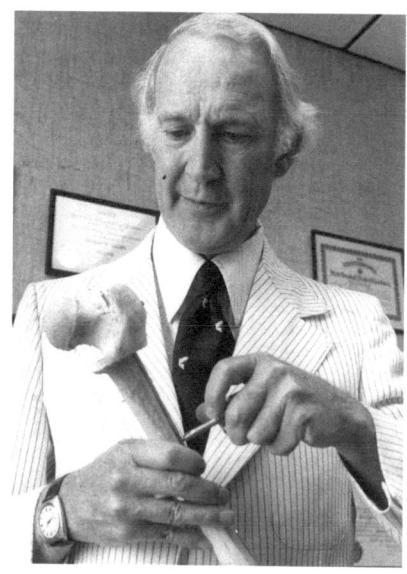

Born:	1923
Died:	2017
Years Active:	50
Location:	Minnesota and Spokane, Washington
Role(s):	Inventor of the first metal cage and a founding architect of Modern Spine Fusion Surgery

Dr. George William Bagby II designed and patented the first metal "cage or basket" to be implanted between two vertebrae to distract the disc space, relieve nerve compression and achieve spinal fusion.

Bagby's device revolutionized spinal surgery by reducing surgical and recovery times for patients. His contributions rank him among the founding architects of modern spine fusion surgery.

The initial Bagby Bone Baskets (BBB) were implanted in horses by George and surgical veterinarian Barrie Grant. The baskets corrected a degenerative spinal disease known as Wobbler's Syndrome, which caused weakness or paralysis in the back legs. The racing and breeding careers of many horses were saved by the BBB and its successor the Kerf Cut Cylinder (KCC). The most famous recipient of the KCC was the Triple Crown winner, Seattle Slew. After many successful surgeries in horses, George teamed with Dr. Stephen Kuslich. They developed and patented the Bagby and Kuslich (BAK) implant for use in humans.

George was born in Waco, Texas on February 7, 1923. His mother, Rita (ne Bolger) was widowed three times and married four. George was ten when his father George Sr. died. Rita remarried and moved George and his sister Caryl (Fenton) to Wheaton, Minnesota. George's stepfather, Jared 'Doc' Burton, a veterinarian, mentored George and inspired him to pursue a medical career.

George attended Temple Medical School in Philadelphia, Pennsylvania as an inactive private in the U.S. Army during World War II. At the war's end he was a general practitioner in Cannon Falls, Minnesota for four years. When the Korean war broke out, Dr. Bagby reenlisted as an Army captain and served as a surgeon at the 171st Evacuation Hospital in Korea.

After the war, Dr. Bagby returned to Minnesota where he trained as an orthopedic surgeon at the Mayo Clinic graduating in 1956. During that time, he designed a self-compressing bone plate for long boned fractures, the first of his many medical inventions.

Inspired by his Texan relatives, who were Southern Baptist missionaries in Brazil, George used the proceeds of his inventions to support many educational institutions. His greatest achievement was to fund the Nalta Hospital in Bangladesh in partnership with Dr. Ruhal Haque and support from local and international Rotarians.

He traveled to the hospital 20 times always accompanied by an amazing team of devoted and talented volunteers. At 83, Dr. Bagby finally retired from medicine but continued over the remaining 11 years of his life to support the Shriner's Hospitals for crippled children and to join Orthopedics Overseas, Spokane South Rotary, Spokane Valley Lions Club and the Unitarian Universalist Church.

Champ Leroy Baker Jr.

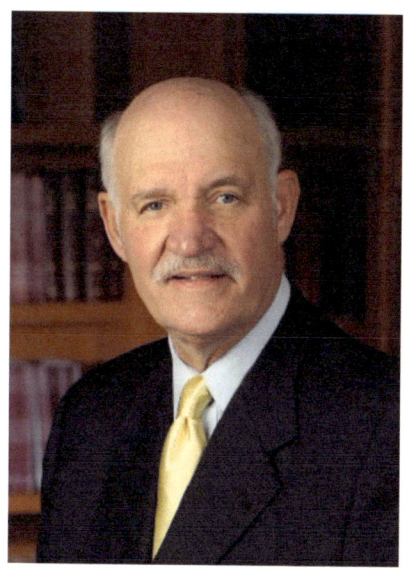

Born:	1946
Died:	2022
Years Active:	30+
Location:	Georgia
Role(s):	Sports Medicine Pioneer, President of Hughston Clinic

Champ Leroy Baker, Jr, was a pioneer in sports medicine. He developed several procedures which are still used today including arthroscopic surgery for tennis elbow and hip bursitis. He was also a significant force at The Hughston Foundation and Clinic.

Dr. Baker served as president of The Hughston Clinic from 1994 to 2000. He was also for a time chair of the Board of Directors of The Hughston Foundation and as program director of the Hughston Sports Medicine Fellowship.

Champ Baker received nearly every prestigious award given by the professional associations and societies to which he belonged. When jokingly asked if receiving all these lifetime achievement awards meant he was 'all washed up', he replied, 'Better to be all washed up with awards than all washed up with no awards.

Baker was an orthopedics professor at Tulane University School of Medicine and at the Medical College of Georgia. He was also active in national and international professional societies including the American Academy of Orthopaedic Surgeons, American Shoulder and Elbow Society, American Orthopaedic Society for Sports Medicine, American Orthopaedic Association, International Society of Arthroscopy, Knee Surgery and Orthopaedic Sports Medicine, and Arthroscopy Association of North America.

He served as president of the American Orthopaedic Society for Sports Medicine, Southern Orthopaedic Association, Georgia Orthopaedic Society, and Georgia Shoulder and Elbow Society. He was inducted into the Halls of Fame of both the Chattahoochee Valley Sports and the American Orthopaedic Society of Sports Medicine.

In 2010, he received the George D. Rovere Award from the American Orthopaedic Society of Sports Medicine for his significant contributions to sports medicine education.

He was also honored with the award Mr. Sports Medicine presented annually by the society to a person who has made significant contribution to sports medicine.

The National Athletic Trainers Association also awarded him with the President's Challenge Award. And the Southern Orthopaedic Association with the Distinguished Southern Orthopaedist Award.

Baker was born in Alexandria, Louisiana, on August 3, 1946, to the late Champ L. Baker, Sr. and Astrid Hiie Baker, a nurse. His mother was his inspiration for his medical career.

At 6'5"tall and an athlete, Champ Baker had hoped to have a career in basketball and played his first year at Louisiana State University. His aspirations, however, changed in his sophomore year when "Pistol Pete" Maravich, who went on to be a professional basketball player, joined the team. Baker continued to support the team throughout the years and found a new passion for sports medicine.

He received both his undergraduate and medical degrees from Louisiana State University. He then joined the U.S. Army and completed his orthopedic residency at Letterman Army Medical Center in San Francisco and Shriners Hospital for Crippled Children in St. Louis.

Baker also did a sports medicine fellowship under Dr. Jack Hughston in Columbus, Georgia in 1979. He retired from the Army as a Lieutenant Colonel in 1982 and joined The Hughston Clinic in 1982 where he remained on staff until his retirement.

Baker's legacy lives on in many ways, but notably in the many medical textbooks and scientific articles he authored. He also served on the editorial board of several medical journals.

His support of athletes never wavered. He was team physician for several local and regional athletic teams, including the University of Alabama and Columbus State University, where he was inducted into their Sports Hall of Fame.

Baker funded scholarships for students in nursing and athletic training and was instrumental in bringing MercyMed to Columbus, providing indigent healthcare to his community. He is also a past-president of the Board of Trustees of Columbus State University and a board member of The Bo Bartlett Center.

Lew Bennett

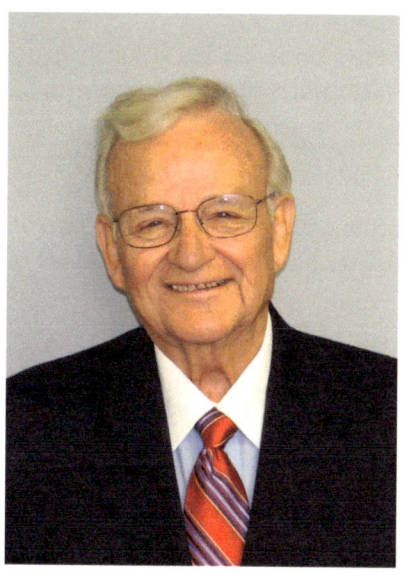

Lew Bennett was one of the founders of Howmet (later Howmedica Corporation, the core of Stryker Corporation's joint arthroplasty business) an instrumental founder and senior executive at Sofamor Danek (now Medtronic Spine), senior executive at Richards Manufacturing (now Smith & Nephew's large joint and sports medicine business), and, finally, senior executive and/or board member for NuVasive, Inc., SpineMedica Corp., Custom Spine, Inc., and HydroCision, Inc.

Lew Bennet was one of the catalysts and most beloved executives that built the practices and business of orthopedic and spine care.

Lew was born in 1926 in Nashville, Tennessee. He attended West High School and went on to marry his grade school sweetheart, Betty Gene Boone, in Nashville in 1947.

One of Lew's first jobs was with a company called Ethicon, Inc, a division of Johnson & Johnson, the largest medical device company in the world. Lew was Salesman of the Year…the rest is orthopedic industry history.

Born:	1926
Died:	2013
Years Active:	50+
Location:	Tennesee
Role(s):	Howmet and Sofamor Danek founder, senior executive and Board Member for numerous orthopedic and spine companies

From his earliest days with J&J, Lew learned to develop personal relationships… not only with key hospital decision makers, but with their secretaries and assistants as well. "Lovable Lew" had his photo affixed to his business card, so everyone would remember him."

Lew created and defined the role of professional medical sales representative.

"Lew brought his experience and positive personality to Smith & Nephew Orthopedics (formerly Richards Medical) in 1980. He helped develop the company's sales organization, as well as organizing teaching seminars on how to manage successful physician practices (with a focus on patient satisfaction). Lew developed strong personal relationships with hundreds of orthopedic surgeons in the U.S. and overseas."

In the more than 50 years that Lew Bennett been a key leader and visionary in the orthopedic and spine worlds he never met a stranger and spoke to everyone with his signature, "Hi, How ya doing?"

When they responded in kind, his answer was always "Like a million!"

Lew held executive positions at multiple orthopedic and spine companies in the industry and developed long-term personal relationships with thousands of surgeons.

As one of the founders of Howmet (which later became Howmedica Corporation), Lew helped position the company for an acquisition by Stryker. Lew also held executive positions at Sofamor Danek (now a division of Medtronic Spine), Richards Manufacturing (now Smith and Nephew), and NuVasive.

His was also CEO of SpineMedica, president of Custom Spine and board member of Hydrocision.

At some point, Lew got the public speaking bug, and he became a popular consultant and presenter, helping many people and surgeon practices. In all, he lectured at over 300 orthopedic and neurological resident programs. In addition, he consulted for over 550 orthopedic and neurological practices and universities.

Randal R. Betz, M.D. of Shriners Hospitals in Philadelphia, remembers, "One of the best years of my life was 1981, when I had the opportunity to meet Lew. At that time, he was giving a new residents program on practice management. Since then, Lew has done several hundred of these, and these were then refined and developed into a program for spine fellows and then into one for practicing physicians."

"During Lew's practice management session, there were several principles he liked to teach. One was "listening and learning."

"Everyone he interviewed could expect to sit there for two hours; on average he checked roughly 12 references. He often said to people, "Why the heck should I hire you?" When I spoke with him a few years ago he told me, "I want the whole story on a person, practically from when they were in diapers. Most distributors I know of don't take the time to thoroughly interview and vet the person. Weeks or months later they're wondering what went wrong."

Lew *lived* a positive attitude. "Look," said Lew, "a negative person is the kind who goes to an orgy and then complains about the cheese dip. Weed out these people."

John McClellan M.D. of the Nebraska Spine Center met Lew Bennett during his orthopedic residency training. He says, "Lew was a great mentor and a true friend. He taught the residents how to evaluate job opportunities to help us find the right position. I later met him when he visited our spine surgical practice. He taught the group how to better manage our practice and helped us run annual retreats."

"He taught us about marriage. He provided us with a book 'Like a Million' that taught me to have frequent discussions with my wife about our individual goals. It helped me build a stronger marriage. He taught life lessons on the golf course when at almost twice my age he could hit the golf ball straighter and shoot a lower score."

"Lew was the world's greatest mentor and a true friend. I will miss my friend."

Ron Pickard, former CEO of Sofamor Danek recalls time with his dear friend: "Lew was one in a million; someone you just enjoyed being around. As Lew would say, 'He wears well with people.' Lew, you certainly did."

Adele Ludin Boskey

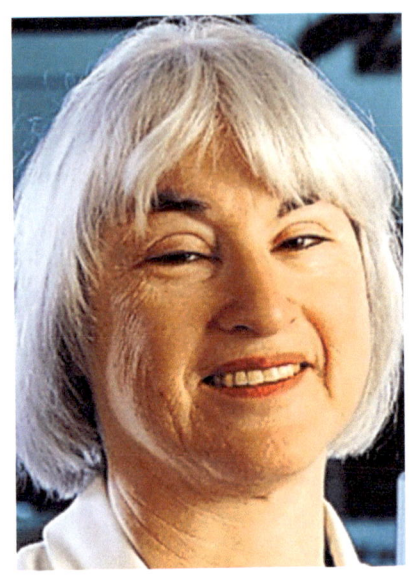

Born:	1943
Died:	2017
Years Active:	45+
Location:	New York City
Role(s):	Senior scientist and program director Musculoskeletal Integrity Program, Starr Chair in Mineralized Tissue Research at the Hospital for Special Surgery

Adele Ludin Boskey, Ph.D., was the first female president of the Orthopaedic Research Society (ORS), Starr Chair in Mineralized Tissue Research, senior scientist, and program chair of the Musculoskeletal Integrity Program at the Hospital for Special Surgery (HSS) in New York City, the preeminent orthopedic teaching hospital in the world.

She was the go-to scientist in the world of bone...and she graced the halls of HSS for 45 years.

Her research was continuously funded by the National Institutes of Health (NIH) and she authored or co-authored 270 seminal articles during her career which were fundamental to building the modern practice of orthopedic and spine care.

Dr. Boskey obtained her bachelor's in chemistry from Barnard College and her Ph.D. from Boston University. She then began her post-doctoral fellowship at the Imperial College in London, completing her fellowship at HSS in 1972.

As a physical chemist Dr. Boskey devoted her career to understanding biomineralization and bone formation. "Her pioneering research in the application of biophysical and imaging technologies to define the composition, structure and functional properties of bone changed the field, greatly deepened our understanding of bone quality and fracture risk and led to the success of the present research programs at HSS. Her foundational research contributed to the understanding of a number of musculoskeletal diseases, including osteoarthritis, osteoporosis, osteogenesis imperfect and growth plate abnormalities." – from her colleagues at HSS.

Lionel Ivashkiv, M.D., chief scientific officer at Hospital for Special Surgery, said of his longtime colleague, "She was one of the real founding scientists and original leaders of research at HSS. She helped to establish the research division back in the '80s and '90s, and without her, we really would not have gotten anywhere near where we are now."

"I think her dedication and hard work were extraordinary, but I also think her spirit of wanting to mentor junior scientists—and these are people from different backgrounds, including orthopedic surgeons, engineers, and a whole slew of students, post-doctoral fellows—this was really something that was important to her and allowed her to have an impact on science, not just at HSS, but across the country and around the world."

"She was the founding scientist and world leader in the investigation of the quality of bone, which is very important in understanding osteoporosis and thinking of new ways to treat it."

"She pioneered a variety of techniques, including biophysical and imaging techniques, to determine if bone has good or poor quality, and how bone quality is related to fracture susceptibility and the ability to recover from injury. This was a big step beyond the thinking at the time, when it was thought that just knowing the amount of bone mineral or density would be enough. She was a visionary and a real giant in the bone field. She was instrumental in driving forward bone research within the orthopedic area."

Dr. Boskey's many awards included the Lawrence G. Raisz Award from the American Society for Bone and Mineral Research, the Distinguished Investigator Award from the ORS/Orthopaedic Research and Education Foundation (OREF) and the Pioneers in Innovation Award and the Women's Leadership Forum Award from the ORS. She also received the ORS/American Orthopaedic Association Alfred R. Shands, Jr. Award.

Mathias Bostrom, M.D., an attending orthopedic surgeon at HSS, knew Dr. Boskey for 27 years.

"She's recognized as a world expert in bone, bone mineralization and how bones were affected by various pharmacological agents. With her background in chemistry, she was a world expert on how bone quality changed with various treatment modalities. People would come from around the world and want her to do the bone analysis because she had such state-of-the-art approaches."

"She was recognized by the Orthopaedic Research Society as one of the leading female mentors in the country. She really wanted to improve not only orthopedic science, but the ability of women in particular to advance their careers in orthopedics and in research in general."

Dr. Bostrom says the key to understanding Dr. Boskey is "her amazing commitment to the next generation of scientists, particularly to orthopedic clinician scientists and also to women orthopedic scientists. Her mentorship was just amazing."

Jane Salmon, M.D., a senior scientist, and Collette Kean Research Chair at HSS, had known Dr. Boskey since 1982, when Dr. Salmon started working in the HSS Research Laboratory as a rheumatology fellow. Dr. Salmon, director, SLE APS (Systemic Lupus Erythematosus- Antiphospholipid) Center of Excellence at HSS, said, "She's always been a person with wisdom AND warmth. A basic scientist who asked clinically derived questions. Dr. Boskey was supportive and understood the challenges of women working in science, as well as the opportunities. She was loving, supportive and nurturing, but with high standards. She was an amazing woman. She was an innovator."

Antonio (Tony) Castellvi

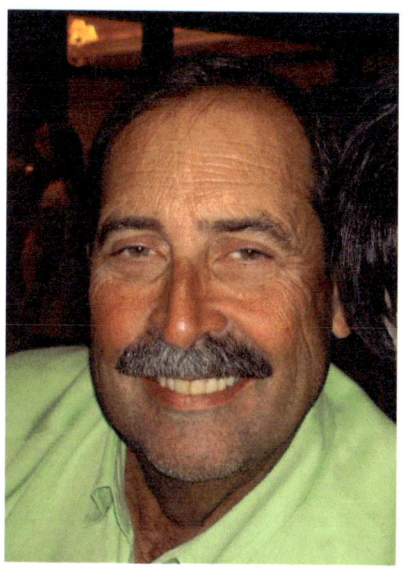

Born:	1953
Died:	2014
Years Active:	30+
Location:	South Florida
Role(s):	Director of Spine Fellowship, Florida Orthopaedic Institute, Founder and Course Chair, Current Solutions in Spine Surgery (now the Castellvi Meeting).

Dr. Antonio (Tony) Castellvi was one of the most influential spine surgeons of the past twenty years. He played a pivotal role through his research and his popular annual course in spine surgery, in expanding the understanding and preserving motion preservation in spine.

His research in spine motion preservation led to numerous publications in both Spanish and English and podium presentations at more than 50 conferences and meetings nationally and internationally.

Dr. Castellvi was an honors graduate of the University of Zaragoza Medical School in Spain and completed his orthopedic residency at the University of South Florida, his spine fellowship at the University of Rochester.

Over the course of more than 30 years, Tony built a very successful practice focusing on cervical, lumbar, or thoracolumbar problems, degenerative disease and deformity, scoliosis, reconstruction, spinal cord injury and motion preservation.

In 2005, Dr. Castellvi founded an innovative educational course which he titled Current Solutions in Spine Surgery and based it in Hawks Cay, Florida. Castellvi's course became instrumental in introducing, debating and, ultimately, understanding advanced spine surgery concepts and approaches.

The meeting became best known as the annual "Duck Key Meeting."

For many spine researchers and practitioners, Dr. Castellvi's meeting was (and remains today) one of the highlights of the year.

Additionally, he served as a board member of the International Society for the Advancement of Spine Surgery and is one of 10 members to review abstracts to determine which will be presented internationally.

Dr. Castellvi was also assistant professor at the University of South Florida and Director of Spine Fellowship at the Florida Orthopaedic Institute.

"Tony was a 'true innovator and thought leader in spine surgery." – Thomas J. Errico MD, Past President, ISASS and Professor, NYU Grossman School of Medicine

"I always thought of Tony as a clinician scientist—meaning he always thought about the patient and his/her outcome from a pragmatic view, yet he grounded everything he did in data and evidence." – Marc Viscogliosi, Partner VB LLC.

"Trained by Lou Goldstein and Don Chan. Tony's key paper was on transitional vertebra which was published in Spine 1984." David Polly MD, Chief of Spine Surgery, University of Minnesota

"Tony's wonderful Duck Key meeting is one of the great and personal favorite spine educational meetings of every year." Richard D Guyer, MD, President, Texas Back Institute

"In addition to his commitment to his patients, Tony was an innovator, involved in the development and study of a number of novel spinal technologies. He was however truly in his element during his annual course in the Keys when he was leading clinical case discussions; challenging us to think critically and at the same time applying his ample common sense to solving clinical challenges." Frank M. Phillips, MD, Professor, Orthopaedic Surgery, Spine Fellowship Co-Director, Rush University Medical Center

"Tony made many important contributions to the spine surgery world, particularly in assessing new operative techniques for the treatment of common spinal disorders." – Chris Bono, Past President of the North American Spine Society, Professor of Spine Surgery, Harvard Medical School

"Tony's achievement of establishing a yearly spine meeting in the Keys of Florida that attracted open dialogue on the progress of Spine Care and Surgery based on Sound Scientific grounds has become a must attend for many of us." – Hansen Yuan, Past President of the North American Spine Society, and former Professor of Orthopaedic and Neurological surgery at SUNY.

John S. Collis Jr.

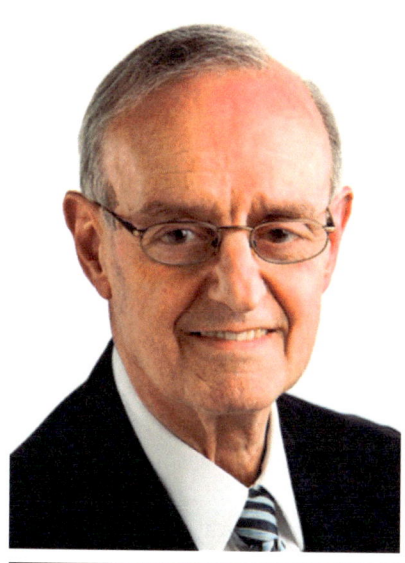

Born:	1931
Died:	2020
Years Active:	50+
Location:	Cleveland, Ohio
Role(s):	Spine surgery pioneer, Director of Spine Surgery at Cleveland Clinic, Director of Neurosurgery Lutheran Hospital and St. Vincent Charity.

John S. Collis was one of the most significant spinal surgery pioneers. Among his many his many first, Dr. Collis was the first neurosurgeon to establish spinal surgery as a neurosurgery sub-specialty. He was also the first physician to treat back pain with corticosteroid injections. He also pioneered many of the anti-infection protocols that are standard of care today.

Dr. Collis was an associate professor at Case Western Reserve University School of Medicine, director of spine surgery at Cleveland Clinic and director of neurosurgery at Lutheran Hospital and St. Vincent Charity Medical Center in Cleveland.

Over the course of his extraordinary career in neurosurgery, which began when he entered practice in 1963 after completing a residency at Cleveland Clinic, John Collis treated 400,000 patients and performed 17,000 spinal surgeries.

Dr. Collis continued to treat patients at St. Vincent's up until six days before his death at age 89.

John S. Collis was born in Lexington, Kentucky, and raised in Winchester, Kentucky, by parents John and Elizabeth. In his youth, he taught Sunday School and played the organ at the Disciples of Christ Church. He was also an Eagle Scout.

He graduated from Saint Agatha's Academy High School in 1947 shortly after turning fifteen. He finished his undergraduate degree at Kentucky Wesleyan College at age eighteen in 1950.

Collis excelled at academics and baseball. In 1949, he was offered a major league contract as a pitcher for the Saint Louis Cardinals. Collis declined in order to focus on pursuing a career in medicine. He graduated from University of Louisville Medical School in 1955 and went on to then complete a neurosurgical residency at the Cleveland Clinic in 1961.

Early neurosurgery focused on head and brain injury, not spine treatment. Dr. Collis saw how common and also how complex back pain and injury were. After 16 years of active medical work at the Clinic, Collis felt there was a dire need for a separate department to specialize in spinal surgery. He thus became the first neurosurgeon to specialize in spinal treatment.

At the time, the medical community did not validate a need for such a specialty. For this reason, Collis chose to go into private practice. Today, many neurosurgeons and orthopedists are spine specialists and over 800,000 spinal surgeries are performed annually.

Donlin M. Long, M.D., former Director of Spinal Surgery at Johns Hopkins Medical Center, spoke of Dr. Collis' accomplishments at a recent celebration of Collis' work. He said, "John's example and success convinced the next generation of neurosurgeons and orthopedic surgeons that spinal surgery was a viable subspecialty. Now the majority of neurosurgeons in practice do mostly spinal surgery… John Collis can take credit for all of this. He was the first to tell us why it was important to emphasize the spine and he then showed us how to do it!"

"I've done about 16,000 major cases; 5,000 of those have been fusions," Dr. Collis stated at a 2017 lifetime achievement award acceptance ceremony in Cleveland. "I've never had my first infection in all those fusions," he said.

Dr. Collis said, "I'd say the aspects of spinal surgery that I have perhaps started, certainly contributed to, is geared about safety for the patient." He described the keys to avoiding infections as: preparation of the body before surgery, antibiotics use and efficient wound draining.

While serving as a military surgeon in Hawaii, Dr. Collis researched infection combat after a series of infections became so rampant it led to the closure of a Hawaiian hospital.

He first instructed patients to take a "septosol shampoo and shower" the night before and morning of surgery.

Secondly, Dr. Collis said he initiated new antibiotics protocols. Dr. Collis stated, "Everyone used antibiotics after you had an infection, but after you had the infection, antibiotics almost can't get to the abscess. You have to open that abscess, drain it, so the antibiotics can get to it."

"I thought, why not have those antibiotics in you before you start the surgery?" he said.

Dr. Collis reported he received initial criticism for "excessive use of antibiotics." However, he proceeded to administer pre-surgery antibiotics after a careful comparison of the risks of excessive antibiotics and the risks of surgical infections.

Pre-surgical baths became protocol by the late 1970s and pre-surgical antibiotics use became standard care in the 1990s "Now, I don't think there's any surgeon in this country who does spinal surgery without preoperative antibiotics," he said. "I'm very proud of that."

Dr. Collis contributed to the invention of various spinal surgery tools and technologies. These surgical instruments included those for total disc replacement, a table for disc puncture testing and treatment, a laminectomy retractor, and various other spinal retractors.

Collis wrote a multitude of publications on spinal surgery topics. In addition, Collis was also an innovator in providing patients with a complete copy of all medical and test records and doctor's notes.

Even during the COVID-19 pandemic, Collis continued to be devoted to his patients, quickly adapting to telemedicine in order to care for patients and confer with surgeons.

"I look at patients like they are family. I believe we must treat others the way we want to be treated," said Dr. Collis. "That is why in my operating room environment is church-like, and I mean the old fashioned church, when it was quiet. At a Catholic Mass, the attention is on the Eucharist, on God; in my operating room I want my team quiet, focused only on the patient."

Collis was active in both his local and the national Greek Orthodox Church, served on the Archdiocese Council for 20 years, served on the Board of Trustees of Hellenic College Holy Cross Greek Orthodox School of Theology and served as chair of fundraising for Saints Constantine and Helen Cathedral in Cleveland Heights and the Hellenic Preservation Society of Northeastern Ohio.

Dr. and Mrs. Collis were also closely involved in the restoration and preservation and restoration of a collection of painted icons from the mid-twentieth century Mount Athos in Greece.

D. Kay Clawson

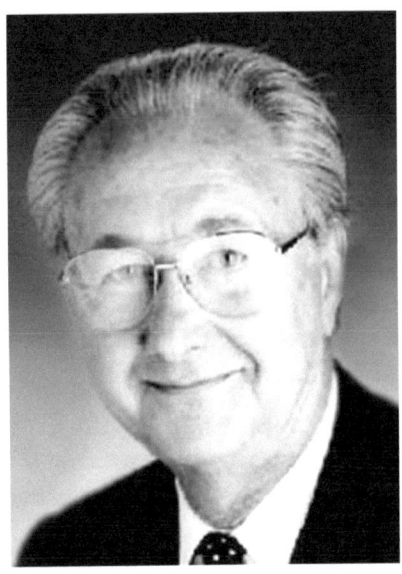

Born:	1928
Died:	2016
Years Active:	40+
Location:	Kentucky
Role(s):	President Association of Bone and Joint Surgeons, Founding member AOSSM, Dean University of Kentucky College of Medicine, Chairman of the Association of American Medical Colleges

D. Kay Clawson, M.D., was a founding member of the American Orthopaedic Society of Sports Medicine, former chairman of the Association of American Medical Colleges, past President of The Association of Bone and Joint Surgeons, founding Chairman of the Department of Orthopaedic Surgery at the University of Washington and dean of the University of Kentucky (UK) College of Medicine from 1975 to 1983.

A Salt Lake City native, Dr. Clawson completed medical school at Harvard University, and his orthopaedic residency at Stanford University. He joined the University of Washington in 1958, and in 1965, he became the founding Chairman of the Department of Orthopaedic Surgery at the school, a position he held for 10 years.

Dr. Clawson served leadership roles in myriad orthopaedic, academic, and organized medicine organizations. He wrote prolifically, and he thoroughly relished his role at the head of the table or behind the podium. He was energetic and moved quickly. As was noted at his retirement, he was a visionary leader who was always out front. In fact, he was often so far out in front that those providing supporting roles could easily lose sight of his next vision.

As a strong leader, he often used both influential national and local contacts to provide linkages to the financial and political resources needed to realize his vision. During his tenure as Dean of the University of Kentucky College of Medicine, Dr. Clawson helped raise funds for additions to the Chandler Medical Center and the School of Medicine. Because of his tireless efforts, University of Kentucky officials renamed a wing of the Kentucky Clinic, which was the primary UK HealthCare outpatient clinic, the "D. Kay Clawson Pavilion." The ceremony took place on his 75th birthday

Among Dr. Clawson's many accomplishments was advancing the educational mission at the University of Kentucky which may well have been his finest achievement. He was the driving force behind that institution's annual New Faculty Development retreats, which were held annually at State Parks throughout Kentucky. These two-day events brought newly hired faculty together in a rural setting that gave individuals a sense of place in Kentucky."

At the retreat, institutional leaders would talk about the mission of the college of medicine and the role of the university as a statewide health care provider.

Each retreat included, naturally, an overview of UK's medical curriculum and sessions specifically focused on the nuts and bolts of teaching, including such often sensitive subjects as promotion and tenure process.

That legacy of openness and collegiality made the University of Kentucky college of medicine one of the finest academic institutions in the United States.

Reflecting the rapid acceleration of orthopedic and medical technique, bioengineering and invention during his tenure as dean, Dr. Clawson nurtured a culture of educational innovation.

Carol L. Elam EdD said this about Dr. Clawson, "He was an incredible leader and visionary. He always had a sense of what he wanted to accomplish...and was able to identify and support the individuals who could help him implement his vision. He knew how to identify the right people to be on his team...and understood the power of teamwork."

"In 1989, he delivered the Chairman's Address at the 100th Annual Meeting of the Association of American Medical Colleges. The Education of the Physician, a paper published in 1990 in Academic Medicine, addresses issues that continue to be pertinent today."

"Dr. Clawson never lost his passion for work... and his desire to influence the next generation of physicians."

"As an Emeritus Professor, he joined the Admissions Committee of UKCOM where he served as a member for 21 years."

"He was inspired by the candidates he interviewed. He was a strong advocate of the applicants who he thought were well prepared in intellect and in passion for the profession."

"For those students who were not quite ready for the challenges of medical education, he offered them encouragement and targeted counseling, helping them to redress their areas of needed improvement."

"Numerous current students and graduates have shared with me that Dr. Clawson supplied them with encouragement and inspiration as they prepared for medical school, and that they were grateful that he shared his wisdom and demonstrated particular care for them as individuals."

Lawrence Douglas Dorr

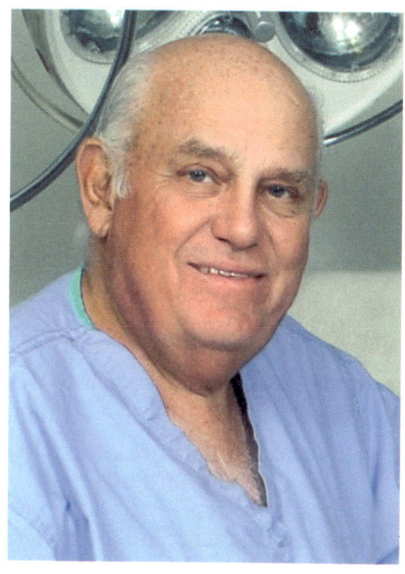

Lawrence Douglas Dorr, M.D., is one of the giants of medicine, founder of The Hip Society and The Knee Society and the driving visionary behind Operation Walk,

Dr. Dorr was born April 13, 1941, in Storm Lake, Iowa. He spent his early life in Iowa and was very proud of his Midwest roots.

He attended graduate school and medical school at University of Iowa and then did an internship at Los Angeles County and University of Southern California Medical Center.

Dr. Dorr also served his country as Lieutenant Commander, United States Navy Medical Corps at Camp Pendleton, California and Jacksonville, Florida from 1967 to 1971.

He then completed his residency in orthopedic surgery at Los Angeles County and University of Southern California Medical Center before starting his fellowship along with Dr. Alan Inglis in joint replacement under Dr. Chitranjan Ranawat at The Hospital for Special Surgery in New York from July 1976 to July 1977.

Born:	1941
Died:	2020
Years Active:	50+
Location:	Los Angeles, California
Role(s):	Founder The Hip Society, The Knee Society and Operation Walk.

Dr. Ranawat, Clinical Professor of Orthopaedic Surgery at Weill Medical College of Cornell University and Attending Orthopaedic Surgeon at HSS, became his mentor and friend and they collaborated many times on a variety of clinical studies, device design, The Hip and Knee Society and other projects.

In 1978, Dr. Dorr became a board certified orthopedic surgeon and started his career in Los Angeles at Los Angeles County and University of Southern California Medical Center and Rancho Los Amigos Hospital in Downey as an attending surgeon.

Dr. Dorr pioneered many of the rapid recovery techniques that are now standard of care for orthopedic patients. His minimally invasive surgical techniques, pain management, the Dorr bone type classification, and his discovery of the relationship of the spinopelvic to the hip has transformed the field of orthopedic care.

Dr. Dorr began designing implants in 1982. His designs for Zimmer's APR stem first came to market in 1984, which were followed by the Apollo knee replacement in the early 1990s.

He was one of the first surgeons to use cementless prosthetic joints. The story goes that he drew one on a napkin in 1982 when out to dinner with Dr. Ranawat.

Dr. Dorr is also one of the founders of The Knee Society and The Hip Society and a member of many orthopedic associations.

It was at a dinner at Dr. Ranawat's house during the 1983 American Academy of Orthopaedic Surgeons Annual Meeting, a time when total knee arthroplasty was becoming a popular treatment for knee arthritis, that the society was first created. His goal was to advance education and research in the area of total knee arthroplasty and arthritis of the knee joint.

He is also the founder of the American Academy of Hip and Knee Surgeons, The Bone and Joint Institute and The Dorr Arthritis Institute, turning Los Angeles into an international destination for joint replacement.

Patients came to him from across the United States and internationally as his reputation grew. He personally trained over 100 clinical and research fellows. The Dorr Bone Classification which he developed in 1993 is often used to categorize bone types prior to hip reconstruction.

Giving back to others was always important to Dr. Dorr as well. After being inspired by Operation Smile which provides free corrective surgery for impoverished children with cleft lips, he started his own nonprofit called Operation Walk in 1996.

The nonprofit organization provides free joint replacement for people in underserved countries and the U.S. Implants, surgical materials medications and recovery equipment are donated by American companies.

He put together a team of surgeons, doctors, nurses and physical therapists who all donated their time to perform the surgeries and to educate local doctors in countries such as Cuba, China, Nepal, Philippines, El Salvador, Tanzania, Guatemala, Nicaragua and Vietnam. Operation Walk has now operated on over 17,000 people.

Over the years, he partnered with Zimmer Biomet, Johnson and Johnson, MAKO, Cardinal Health and Medline. He published hundreds of peer-reviewed manuscripts, book chapters and books on the practice of total joint replacement.

In the 2000s, he helped develop computer technology to improve hip and knee replacement. He retired from Keck Medical Center of USC in June 2019.

Lowry Barnes, M.D., the 30th president of the American Association of Hip and Knee Surgeons said, "Isaac Newton popularized 'If I have seen further, it is by standing on the shoulders of giants' in reference to his advancement of science."

"Truly, Larry Dorr was a giant in the field of hip and knee arthroplasty. Many of us "have seen more" and accomplished more because of his example and mentoring."

"He was a giant in the development of some of our most significant hip and knee organizations. In addition to being a founding member of the American Association of Hip Knee surgeons, he was also a founding member of The Hip Society and Knee Society. He clearly saw the benefit of academic fellowship and the idea of peers pushing peers to do more and more in their field of expertise."

"Despite his many impressive academic contributions related to techniques of hip and knee arthroplasty, he will always be remembered as a giant in the world of philanthropy and service to others."

"He founded Operation Walk, and many patients across the world are walking pain free now because of this organization and its mission to make joint replacement available to those who do not otherwise have access to these remarkable life-changing procedures. The leaders of the many chapters of Operation Walk across our country who continue to provide this service across the world stood on Larry's shoulders to see the future and what they could do to help others."

Former Zimmer Biomet CEO Ray Elliott said, "The mile wide smile and the inevitable rib crushing bear hug were not only a part of our ritual but a reflection of the big heart that came with Larry Dorr. Somehow the day just got a lot better courtesy of the proud Storm Lake Iowan that made it to the very top of his profession, trained so many, gave back endlessly through Operation Walk and other philanthropies but never forgot who he was...and nor will we ever forget our business partner and friend."

A. Seth Greenwald, D. Phil (Oxon), director of Orthopaedic Research Laboratories and founder of Current Concepts in Joint Replacement, said, "Larry Dorr was a larger than life character whose no nonsense approach to accepting nothing less than excellence in hip and knee reconstruction was his mantra. I will always count Larry as a friend and stand-up colleague who, both in his personal practice and through the founding of Operation Walk, continues to bring arthritic relief to thousands of patients around the world who otherwise might have been excluded from the best of orthopedic healthcare. Larry's contributions to the orthopedic peer-reviewed literature, his dedication to educate through the Masters' meetings as well as his ability and imagination to characterize life's experiences as a novelist all define an individual who has made his mark."

Dorr's awards include a Distinguished Alumni Award from Cornell College (2003) and University of Iowa Carver College of Medicine (2006), Humanitarian Award from American Academy of Orthopaedic surgeons (2005), Humanitarian of the Year Award from the Iowa Orthopedic Society (2007), American Academy of Hip and Knee Surgeons Humanitarian of the Year Award (2017) and Honorary Member of the Cuban Orthopedic Society (2019).

William F. Enneking

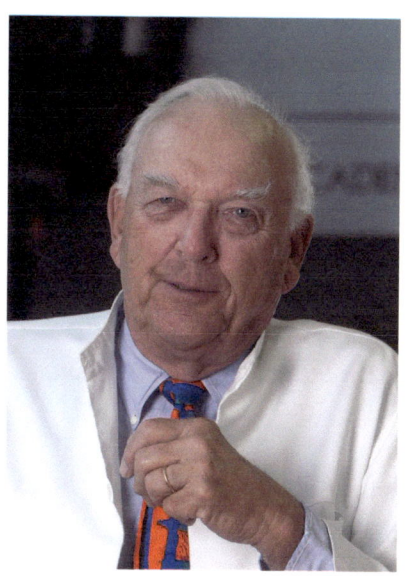

Born:	1926
Died:	2014
Years Active:	40+
Location:	Florida
Role(s):	Co-founder University of Florida College of Medicine, Chief of Surgery University of Mississippi and the first Chair of the Department of Orthopedics and Rehabilitation University of Florida.

Dr. William F. Enneking was a co-founder of the University of Florida College of Medicine, the first chief of orthopedic medicine at the University of Florida College of Medicine and the first chair of the Department of Orthopedics and Rehabilitation.

Born in Madison, Wisconsin in 1926, Dr. Enneking earned his M.D. at the University of Wisconsin in 1949, and then interned at the University of Colorado for one year. From 1952-55 he completed an orthopedic residency at the University of Chicago.

He spent nine years in the U.S. Navy (1943-1952) and in 1955 became an Instructor in orthopedics at the University of Chicago.

In 1956 he moved on to the University of Mississippi where he served as Associate Professor of Surgery and Chief of Orthopedic Surgery. The remainder of his stellar career was spent at the University of Florida, where served as chair from 1974-1980.

Mark Scarborough, M.D., the William F. Enneking, William E. Anspach and Orthopedic Alumni Chair in the College of Medicine Department of Orthopedics and Rehabilitation at the University of Florida said this of his father-in-law, "He thought it was exciting to be part of a new medical school and he delighted in educating young medical students to be great physicians. He always said you can train monkeys, but you educate doctors."

Dr. Enneking was a founding member and past president of the International

Limb Salvage Society. "Dr. Enneking was at the forefront of limb salvage surgery. Prior to his era, most patients with malignant bone tumors underwent amputation. He developed much of the cognitive framework that guides the field of musculoskeletal oncology today."

Dr. Enneking was also a past president of the Orthopedic Research Society, the American Board of Orthopedic Surgery, and the American Orthopedic Association.

Dempsey Springfield, M.D. said, "Dr. Enneking was the classic academic physician triple threat. He was a scientist, clinician, and educator. He advanced the science of bone biology and provided extraordinary personal innovative care to thousands of patients, but it was his teaching that most affected those who were around him. He saw educational opportunities in every activity."

"Dr. Enneking knew the sweet spot between the Socratic method and humiliation better than anyone."

Albert B Ferguson Jr

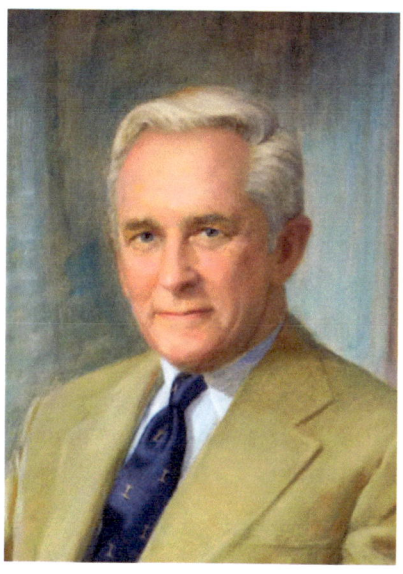

Born:	1919
Died:	2014
Years Active:	43
Location:	Florida
Role(s):	Founder of the University of Pittsburgh Department of Orthopedic Surgery, founding member Hip Society, former President American Board of Orthopedic Surgery

Albert B. Ferguson founded the University of Pittsburgh Department of Orthopedic Surgery in 1954.

He also was an honorary fellow of the British Orthopedic Association and the Japanese Orthopedic Society. He was also, at one time, president of the American Orthopedic Association, a founding member of the Hip Society, and president of the American Board of Orthopedic Surgery.

Dr. Ferguson, born in New York City on June 10, 1919, did his undergraduate work at Dartmouth College and then went on to graduate from Harvard Medical School in 1943.

Albert Ferguson served three years as United States Marine in the Pacific Theater during World War II.

After the war, Dr. Ferguson trained in surgery and orthopedic surgery at Boston's Children's, Peter Bent Brigham, and Massachusetts General Hospitals. It was in 1953 that he took the helm at "Pitt" being appointed the Silver Professor of Orthopedic Surgery and Chairman of Orthopedic Surgery at the University of Pittsburgh. He remained there until his retirement in 1986.

Dr. Ferguson served as president of various orthopedic organizations, and eventually British and Japanese orthopedic associations would honor him. In 2006, the American Orthopedic Association honored him, and then their Pennsylvania Medical Society gave him the Distinguished Service Award in 2007.

Freddie Fu, M.D., founder of the University of Pittsburgh's sports medicine program, said this about Dr. Ferguson. "He was a surgeon among surgeons who trained 50 leaders in the field. He was able to motivate people by serving as a role model...and he never had to raise his voice."

"He was a great thinker and succeeded in recruited the best people, such as Henry Mankin and Harry Rubash, who both went on to lead Massachusetts General Hospital."

"Dr. Ferguson was direct, but he never put anyone down or was discouraging. He was very positive and encouraging. For example, in grand rounds if someone's paper was not up to par, he never made that person feel bad. Other faculty would have eaten that person for lunch, Dr. Ferguson found a way to make it a win/win situation so that the person would do better next time. He was very unique in that—and many—ways."

Gary Ferguson M.D., Albert Ferguson's son, recalled his father's work ethic. "He got out of bed and attacked the day. He didn't live the days of his life, he attacked them. At age six I lacerated my hand. I was in too much of a hurry to get through a storm door."

"My distraught mother brought me to his office with my hand wrapped in her favorite bathroom towel. At about 6:00 in the evening he was exhausted from a day of seeing patients, all of whom were children at the time. He then had to face a blood-soaked towel around his son's hand as an unexpected last patient."

"We had a longstanding game we played where I would throw a towel in his face as a distraction, and then try to run around him before he could grab me. So now taking in this scene in his office, he grabbed a near-by pillow, threw it in my face, ran around me, and I giggled. I got the role reversal, he put me on the table, sewed up my laceration, and we were good to go."

"My father's credo was that actions are necessary, words are not. Work hard, do the right thing, and the rest will take care of itself."

"And while my dad's colleagues know this already, I'll say it anyway because they all understand how deeply true it is. He loved his colleagues as he loved his sons, daughter, and wife. He would do anything for any colleague. His mission was to make sure everyone was OK. He was relentless in this pursuit."

Freddie Fu

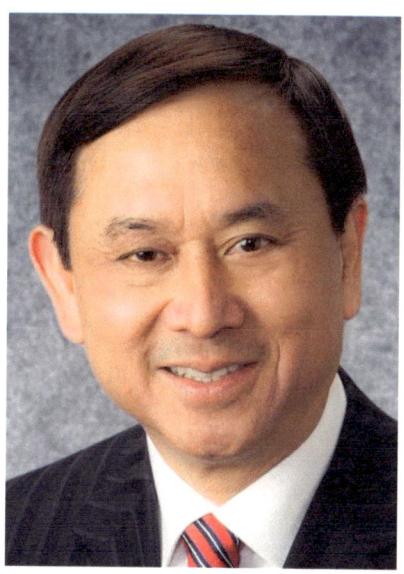

Born:	1951
Died:	2021
Years Active:	46
Location:	Pittsburgh, Pennsylvania
Role(s):	Founder of the University of Pittsburgh Sports Medicine Program, Chair of Orthopedic Surgery UPMC

Freddie Fu, M.D., was internationally revered orthopedic surgeon and founder of the University of Pittsburgh Medical Center's sports medicine program.

Dr. Fu was a leading global expert in ACL reconstruction, a prolific medical author and editor, the company physician for the Pittsburgh Ballet Theatre, as well as the head team physician for the University of Pittsburgh athletic department.

"A pioneer in modern/future surgery. A leader who helped transform Pittsburgh's economy to eds & meds." Pittsburgh Mayor Bill Pedutohe wrote on Twitter.

A native of Hong Kong, Dr. Fu immigrated to the U.S. in the 1970s at age 18, to study at Dartmouth College. While there, he was active in Chinese and International student associations and played on the champion ping pong team. In 1974, he earned an undergrad biology degree at Dartmouth and in 1975 he earned a Bachelor of Medical Studies from Dartmouth's Medical School.

Dr. Fu went on to earn his medical degree from the University of Pittsburgh School of Medicine in 1977. He completed a general surgery internship at Brown University before returning to the University of Pittsburgh for an ortho research fellowship and residency training.

In 1982, he became the chair of the orthopedic surgery department. Dr. Fu founded the first sports medicine program in western Pennsylvania in 1986, subsequently advancing and expanding the UPMC sports medicine program. By 1997, Fu was named orthopaedic surgery department chair.

"Freddie Fu and I met the first day of classes at DMS almost 50 years ago. Like all of us, he seemed anxious, but excited to finally start medical school. Freddie never lost that spark- the enthusiasm and love for learning, and later for research and teaching," said former classmate Oglesby H. Young, M.D., Clinical Assistant Professor of Obstetrics and Gynecology, at Geisel School of Medicine.

Dr. Fu pioneered a variety of arthroscopic surgical techniques for the treatment of shoulder and knee injuries. He initiated extensive knee joint research, studying biomechanics, comparative anatomy, in vivo kinematics and stem cell and regenerative medicine related to the knee.

He published 173 book chapters, over 675 peer-reviewed articles, and edited 30 orthopedic textbooks on sports injury medicine. He was the recipient of over 260 professional awards and honors over the course of his long and expansive career.

At the time of his passing in 2021, Fu's team had over 100 studies on anatomy and evolution of the knee joint in process.

Dr. Fu was the first orthopedic surgeon to conceptualize opting out of one-size-fits-all ACL tear surgery, suggesting instead a more detailed and effective individualized surgical process.

"When we started doing a lot of these it was almost like McDonald's where every one of them was done the same way," he said. "But as I began to do more research… it became clear that…every injury is unique, and every surgery should be unique."

Through his long-term academic and team doctor experience at Pitt, Fu grew in notoriety and went on to treat many high-profile athletes. Through his work as company physician for the Pittsburgh Ballet Theatre, he also treated renowned dancers.

In 2017, famed soccer player Zlatan Ibrahimovic tore his ligament during the return of the Europa League semi-final. The 35-year-old thought he might not ever play the sport again. "Zlatan Ibrahimovic will play for many more years," said Fu after operating on Ibrahimovic. His prediction was accurate.

Dr. Fu's roster of famous patients included: Dan Marino, Jerome Bettis, Joe Namath and Larry Fitzgerald, former Pittsburgh Pirate Andrew McCutchen, and ballet superstar Mikhail Baryshnikov.

Under Dr. Fu's direction, the sports medicine program at Pittsburgh University has become one of the top clinical-research programs and sports medicine training sites in the world. Dr. Fu also helped design and implement the 60-acre UPMC Rooney Sports Complex in 2000. The complex features outdoor and indoor training facilities for the Pittsburgh Steelers and University teams, a fitness center, concussion center and sports medicine research and rehabilitation facilities.

In 2018, the complex medical building was renamed the UPMC Freddie Fu Sports Medicine Center. The practice and training center built in 2015 for the Pittsburgh Penguins, the UPMC Lemieux Sports Complex in Cranberry, was modeled after the complex.

Patients treated at the Complex include Steelers, Pirates, Penguins, five-time Tour de France winner Miguel Indurain and ballet legend Mikhail Baryshnikov.

Dr. Fu was also active with the Pittsburgh Ballet Theatre, the Pittsburgh Symphony, and other arts organizations. In addition to being the Ballet Company physician, he also served on its board of directors. Fu assisted in designing the Benedum Center for the Performing Arts floor in the late 1980s. The "sprung" stage floor helps reduce dancers' injuries. "Because of Dr. Fu, my career was saved. I had an injury at that point in 1986 that people in my position, with what I had to do physically, didn't always recover enough to continue on with their career," said dancer Joe Briggs of the Pittsburgh Ballet.

For many years, Fu commuted through the busy streets of Pittsburgh by bicycle. Dr. Anthony DiGioia, M.D., medical director of the bone and joint center at UPMC Magee Women's Hospital and an ortho colleague who met Fu in the early 1980s, described him as "a tornado of energy all the time. "It was unusual for a physician to be involved in research then," said DiGioia. "He came in like a tornado talking about projects and getting things done. That energy carried through with his work as a clinician and researcher."

James D. Kang, M.D., Thornhill Family Professor of Orthopaedic Surgery and Chair, Department of Orthopaedic Surgery at Brigham and Woman's Hospital, said of Dr. Fu "I worked with Dr. Fu as a resident, then as a faculty colleague, and then as his Vice Chair of the Department at UPMC, before I moved to Boston to become Chair of Orthopaedics at the Brigham. I lived through his entire vision of conceptualizing the UPMC Center for Sports Medicine from its inception to what it has become over a 30-year span."

"Although Dr. Fu was a true visionary, his greatest gift was that he had near photographic memory of everyone he ever met and got to know a special little bit of information about you that he could recall years later. This endearing trait made many patients and colleagues feel special when they were with Dr. Fu."

"Dr. Fu shaped my career, and many of us owe a huge debt of gratitude for his part in enabling our collective success."

David S. Jevsevar, M.D., M.B.A., the chair of Orthopaedics at Geisel School of Medicine and Dartmouth-Hitchcock Medical Center, said of Dr. Fu, "Most importantly in his career, he broke down the barriers against diversity within orthopaedics. He again didn't have to do it, but he knew he was uniquely successful and respected and had the opportunity to do so."

"Freddie's academic progeny led orthopedics in virtually every country in the world. His leadership in [diversity, equity and inclusion] in orthopedics especially for women was unparalleled. Freddie walked the walk," tweeted clinical researcher Lynn Snyder-Mackler.

"I have a good attitude about everything," Dr. Fu said in 2002. "I practice medicine with unconditional love, the way you are with your children. You don't expect anything back. But it does come back to you."

John Samuel Gould

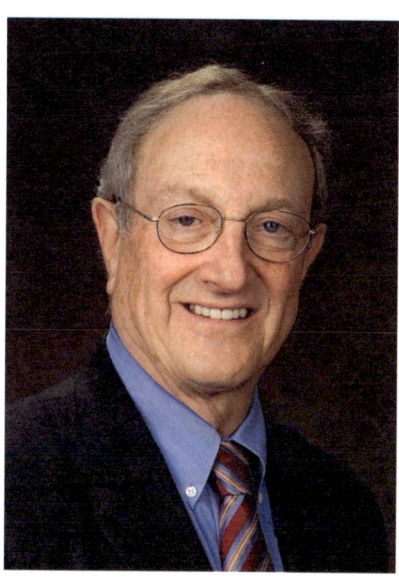

Born:	1939
Died:	2015
Years Active:	45+
Location:	Alabama and Wisconsin
Role(s):	Professor Emeritus University of Alabama at Birmingham, Chief of the Hand Section, Chief of the Department of Orthopaedic Surgery Medical College of Wisconsin. Editor in Chief of Numerous Orthopaedic Journals.

John Samuel Gould was Professor of Surgery at the University of Alabama at Birmingham and, later, Chief of the Department of Orthopaedic Surgery at the Medical College of Wisconsin in Milwaukee.

John Gould was born in St. Johnsbury, Vermont, on May 10, 1939. He graduated from Harvard University in Cambridge, Massachusetts, and in 1964 from the University of Vermont Medical School in Burlington.

Dr. Gould began his general surgery internship at Boston City Hospital, also in 1964. At the completion of his internship and one more year of During the Vietnam War years, Dr. Gould enlisted in the U.S. Navy and was stationed in San Diego, California.

During the first year of his two-year deployment, Dr. Gould served as medical officer aboard the guided missile cruiser USS Canberra, which was deployed to Vietnam. After his time in the Navy, Dr. Gould became a resident in orthopedic surgery at the University of Pittsburgh.

He then joined his father in private practice in Brockton, Massachusetts, for three years, after which time he decided to specialize in orthopedic hand surgery, and began a fellowship at Duke University in Durham, North Carolina.

Dr. Gould was selected to be full Professor of Surgery at University of Alabama Birmingham (UAB) in 1982. He remained chief of the Hand Section until 1986. He was then recruited to be Chief of The Department of Orthopaedic Surgery at the Medical College of Wisconsin.

During his time in Milwaukee, he began to change his focus from hand surgery to surgery of the foot and ankle and instituted a fellowship for orthopedic foot and ankle surgery at the Medical College. He headed that orthopedic program for 10 years before deciding to return to the warmer winters in Birmingham to join Alabama Sports Medicine and Orthopaedic Center until 2004. Dr. Gould then joined Orthopaedic Specialists of Alabama at Baptist Montclair Hospital.

In 2006 he rejoined UAB, this time as Chief of the Foot and Ankle Section of the Orthopaedic Division. There he treated hand and foot and ankle patients, with a special interest in nerve problems and total joint replacement for arthritic ankles. He was awarded the title Professor Emeritus of the UAB School of Medicine by the Board of Trustees on November 7, 2014.

At various times in his career Dr. Gould has been President of the American Orthopaedic Foot and Ankle Society, of the Clinical Orthopaedic Society, of the Mid-America Orthopaedic Association and of the Alabama Orthopaedic Society.

Dr. Gould was also Editor in Chief of the journal, Microsurgery (1986-1996), the American Journal of Orthopaedics (1996-2006), Foot and Ankle Editor for Orthopaedic Knowledge Online Journal, and authored four professional books: 'The Foot Book' Williams and Wilkins, 1988; 'Operative Foot Surgery' W.B. Saunders, 1994; 'My First Love: The Art, The Practice, and The Ethics of Medicine' Seacoast Publishers, 2004; and 'The Handbook of Foot and Ankle Surgery: An Intellectual Approach to Complex Problems' Jaypee Bros. 2013. He also self-published 'The Medical College of Wisconsin: The Gould Years' where he described his ten years as chief of that department.

"John was gifted with a brilliant intellect and ability to organize and train a team of physicians (residents, fellows, nurses) to provide quality care. Over 40 years John has trained a very large number of hand and later foot surgeons. I suspect most of his fellows and residents would attest to his teaching or mentoring skills and would place or rank him number one in this skill set."

Frank Gunston

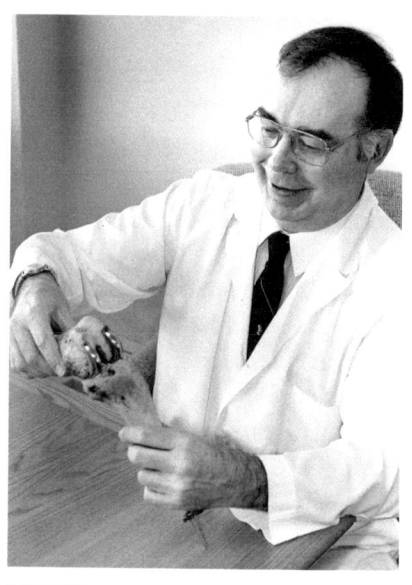

Born:	1934
Died:	2016
Years Active:	40+
Location:	Manitoba, Canada
Role(s):	Pioneering inventor of total knee implant and arthroplasty, winner of the Principal Manning Award for Innovation, Distinguished Surgeon award from the Canadian Orthopaedic Association

Frank Gunston, M.D., an engineer turned surgeon, designed, and developed a revolutionary total knee prosthesis while pursuing a postgrad medical education in England.

Dr. Gunston's contributions and achievements are manifold, and they include the McLaughlin Travelling Fellowship (Sweden and Finland, 1971-72), Assistant Professorship (Surgery, Orthopaedics) at the University of Manitoba Faculty of Medicine, active appointments at Winnipeg General Hospital, the Children's Centre, the Manitoba Rehab Hospital, and later practice in orthopedics and joint replacement at Brandon General Hospital.

Dr. Gunston was awarded the Principal Manning Award for Innovation (1989) for the knee prosthesis, was named Distinguished Surgeon by the Canadian Orthopaedic Association (1994), received the Order of Canada (1997), and the Manitoba Medical Association Scholastic Award (1998). Following his retirement in 2000, he also received the Queen's Golden Jubilee Medal in 2002, and the Diamond Jubilee Medal in 2012.

Dr. Gunston was born in Flin Flon, Manitoba, in 1934 but grew up in Brandon.

He attended and graduated with an engineering degree from the University of Manitoba in 1957, followed by a medical degree in 1963.

Dr. Gunston's total knee prosthesis became a standard of care in the early

1970's. According to Peter MacDonald, M.D. past president of the Canadian Orthopedic Association; "The design has morphed into more modern designs. But certainly Dr. Gunston opened the pathway and set the stage for the modern designs."

Dr. Gunston retired in 2000 after spending the later years of his career practicing in orthopedics and joint replacement at Brandon General Hospital.

Dr. MacDonald, Gibson Professor and Head Section of Orthopaedics, University of Manitoba said; "He was a brilliant man who studied engineering then worked under Sir John Charnley in the United Kingdom (who designed and implanted the first low friction total hip arthroplasty that was successful). He then returned to Canada and designed the polycentric knee which was the first successful total knee design. Since he did not patent it he did not get the credit that he deserved. He was a humble man and did not care for credit or fame. He went on to move from the University of Manitoba into private practice in Brandon, Manitoba, where he finished his career. He continued in later years to try to use his total knee by manufacturing it in his garage. In later years he eventually got recognition for his tremendous contributions!"

Harry N. Herkowitz

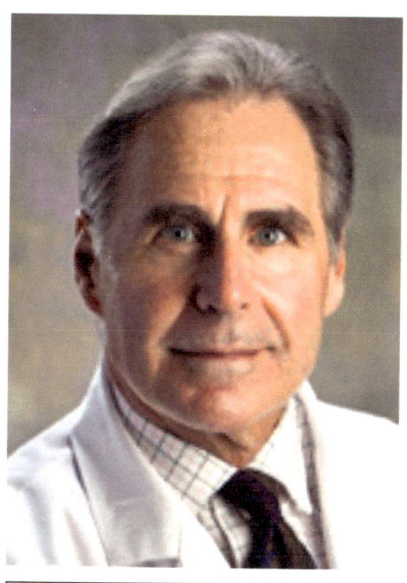

Born:	1948
Died:	2013
Years Active:	40+
Location:	Detroit, Michigan
Role(s):	Pioneer Spine Surgeon, Chairman of Orthopedic Surgery, Beaumont Hospital, Royal Oak, Michigan, President of the Cervical Research Society and the International Society for the Study of Lumbar Spine, and President of the American Board of Orthopaedic Surgery

Harry N. Herkowitz, M.D., was chairman of Orthopaedic Surgery at Beaumont Hospital in Royal Oak, Michigan, president of the Cervical Spine Research Society, the International Society for the Study of the Lumbar Spine, and the American Board of Orthopaedic Surgery.

Dr. Herkowitz came to Beaumont in 1975 for his orthopaedic residency, followed by a fellowship in spine surgery which established his specialty and the focus of his career for the next three decades. He became chairman of the department of Orthopaedic Surgery in 1991 and directed the spine surgery fellowship program from 1987 to 2008.

Dr. Herkowitz's talents and leadership led him to the presidency of the Cervical Spine Research Society, the International Society for the Study of the Lumbar Spine and the American Board of Orthopaedic Surgery.

Dr. Herkowitz's research legacies include contributions to degenerative solutions to aging discs and improving spinal implants. He gained renown with his 1991 landmark study on the treatment of degenerative spondylolisthesis, work which continues to influence current research.

Dr. Herkowitz edited a dozen major textbooks on the spine and served as editor or on the editorial board of major orthopedic and spine journals.

He was a graduate of Wayne State University School of Medicine, did his residency at Beaumont, and completed a spine surgery fellowship at Pennsylvania Hospital in Philadelphia.

Dr. Herkowitz was honored with an Outstanding Academic Excellence Award by Beaumont in 2011. He was also named among the 100 Best Spine Surgeons in America, recognized by Best Doctors in America, and was twice honored with the Volvo Award for Clinical Research in Low Back Pain.

Steve Garfin, M.D., chair of the department of orthopedic surgery at the University of California, San Diego, said of Dr. Herkowitz; "He was a surgeon's surgeon, leader's leader and a clinical scientist's clinical scientist."

Todd Albert, M.D. former president of the Rothman Institute in Philadelphia and former chair of the Department of Orthopaedic Surgery at Thomas Jefferson University said; "Harry Herkowitz was an icon in orthopaedic surgery. He created sentinel scientific works on the treatment of degenerative spondylolisthesis and degenerative cervical disease. He was a leader in multiple societies and on the American Board of Orthopaedic Surgery. Most importantly he was a thread that bound together a great tradition of those trained by Dick Rothman and their progeny."

John Heller, M.D. professor of orthopedic surgery at Emory University said; "Dr. Herkowitz changed the course of contemporary spine surgery through his research, his service to the American Board of Orthopaedic Surgery and leadership in numerous other professional organizations. He was about paying forward the principles and behaviors of his primary mentor, Richard Rothman."

David S. Hungerford

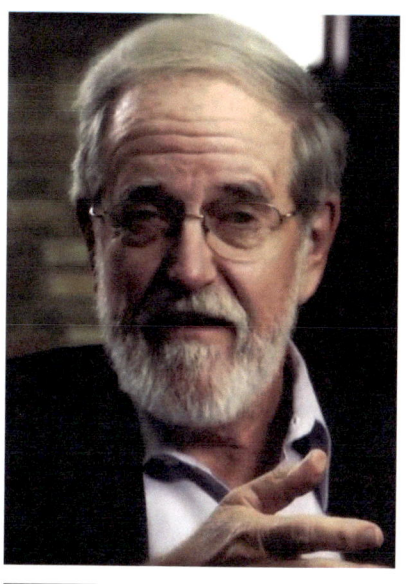

Born:	1939
Died:	2019
Years Active:	
Location:	Baltimore, Maryland
Role(s):	Pioneering Joint Arthroplasty surgeon, Winner of the AAOS Humanitarian award, Chief of Johns Hopkins Scoliosis Clinic, Founding Member of AAHKS, 1st Editor in Chief Journal of Arthroplasty

David S. Hungerford, M.D., had the great good fortune to be trained at the Nuffield Orthopaedic Centre in Oxford, England at precisely the moment that joint arthroplasty emerging as a viable and reliable treatment for end-stage joint arthritis.

Nuffield was the center of the large joint revolution in England in the mid-1960s, before it moved into Europe and the United States. Dr. Hungerford's grounding in large joint arthroplasty came when its basic principles and concepts were being formed.

Dr. Hungerford would later become chief of the division of arthritis surgery at Johns Hopkins University School of Medicine. He established an orthopedic surgery practice at the Good Samaritan Hospital in Baltimore, Maryland, where he led his team as the chief of orthopedic surgery. And he was appointed full professor at Johns Hopkins in 1986.

Hungerford was born in Rochester, New York, to Samuel Hungerford, a school principal and his wife, Marjorie, and then raised in Sodus, New York. It was a serious burn injury as a child that inspired him to become a doctor.

After receiving a bachelor's degree from Colgate University, he studied neurophysiology at the Institut Claude Bernard in Paris as a U.S. Public Health Service postgraduate fellow.

And then back in the U.S., he earned his medical degree at the University of Rochester School of Medicine and completed an internship and surgical residency at Strong Memorial Hospital at the University of Rochester.

Between 1966 and 1969, while with the Army Medical Corps, he worked in Germany, and also performed orthopedic surgery at the Nuffield Orthopaedic Centre in Oxford, England.

Hungerford first joined the Johns Hopkins Hospital in 1972 as a resident in orthopedic surgery.

Good Samaritan Hospital's President Brad Chambers said; Dr. David Hungerford was a pioneer for innovation in orthopedic surgery, developing a porous-coated anatomic artificial knee replacement with medical engineer, Robert Kenna. The technology enabled patients to grow bone cells that fit with their prosthesis and provided better mobility."

"Dr. Hungerford left a tremendous legacy at MedStar Good Samaritan Hospital. His life-long desire to relieve suffering prompted him to continually seek new treatment methods and investigate innovative ways to bring healing and comfort to his patients."

Hungerford specialized in primary hip and knee joint replacements, complex revision surgeries, diagnosis and treatment of osteonecrosis and cartilage regeneration. The field of orthopedic surgery has grown and evolved in so many ways since he first became an orthopedic surgeon and his contributions have helped shaped it to what it is today, especially with regard to hip and knee replacement surgery.

He made significant contributions to the study of core decompression, and on the function and mechanics of the patellar femoral joint.

Hungerford and Robert Kenna, a medical engineer, together developed and produced a universal instrumentation system for use in knee replacement surgery.

To help further innovation in joint replacement, Hungerford became a founding member of the American Association of Hip and Knee Surgeons and was the first editor-in-chief of the *Journal of Arthroplasty* at a time when hip and knee arthroplasty were still fledgling areas of research.

"Dave saw a need for a hip and knee arthroplasty-focused journal when the field and the study of the field was tremendously expanding in the 1980s. He carried out his vision by starting the *Journal* out of his office at the Good Samaritan Hospital in Baltimore. He gave all rights of administering the *Journal* to the [American Association of Hip and Knee Surgeons] in 1990 when we started the organization so we could call this already established journal 'The Official Journal of AAHKS,'" John J. Callaghan, M.D., *Journal of Arthroplasty* editor–in-chief said in a statement.

While he retired from both Johns Hopkins and Good Samaritan in 2011 after

38 years of service, Hungerford continued to play a significant role in orthopedic surgery and in missionary work. In 2013, he received the Humanitarian Award from the American Academy of Orthopaedic Surgeons for his outstanding humanitarian service.

The Chair in orthopedic surgery at Johns Hopkins School of Medicine was officially named for John Hungerford in 2000. He was also named professor emeritus by the Hopkins University Board of Trustees in 2014.

A. Seth Greenwald, DPhil (Oxon), founder of Current Concepts in Joint Replacement meetings and president of Orthopaedic Research Laboratories met Hungerford at the end of 1968 as he was coming to Oxford University as part of his military service, and he will never forget how passionately Hungerford shared all the nuances of orthopedic surgery with him.

"He even bought me a recorder at the PX to record it all. I still have it."

Greenwald said that Hungerford both as a surgeon and teacher contributed so much to the orthopedics community.

Jay Khanna, M.D., an orthopedic spine surgeon at Johns Hopkins said of Hungerford; "He was a gifted surgeon and physician and more importantly a gifted educator. He taught the science and art of orthopaedic surgery, and always emphasized the doctor-patient relationship and its importance in the overall care of a patient.

Hungerford was a member of CURE International, a Christian nonprofit dedicated to providing medical care to children suffering primarily from orthopedic and neurological conditions, he trained orthopedic surgeons throughout Africa to treat various conditions like clubfoot, bowed legs and cleft lips. He also helped create hospitals in Latin America, Africa, the Middle East and the Caribbean which have gone on to treat countless underprivileged patients with advanced diseases of the musculoskeletal system.

He, his wife and kids developed The Tree of Life Foundation which offered financial support to small-scale entrepreneurs in Third World Countries. Hungerford funded it with the royalties from his medical patents.

From 1996 to 2008, he served as chairman of the board of Medical Assistance Programs (MAP), an organization that promotes the total health of people living in developing countries, and in 2009, Hungerford along with his wife Heide started A Common Path Alliance (CPA), an organization that promotes reconciliation between Muslims and Christians. CPA is now TRAC5.

He even co-authored "The Qur'an – with References to the Bible, A Contemporary Understanding," a modern English translation of the Qur'an with more than 3,000 parallel references to the Bible.

Frank Jobe

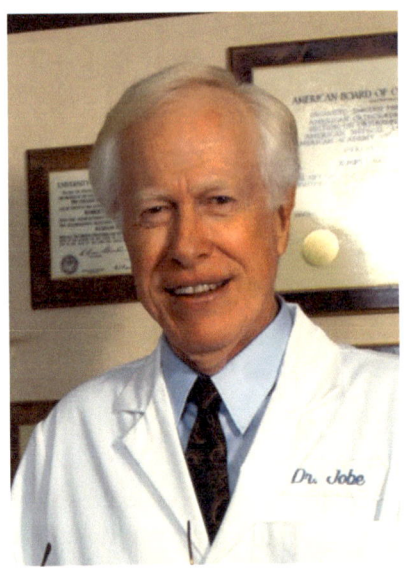

Born:	1925
Died:	2014
Years Active:	40+
Location:	Santa Monica, California
Role(s):	Arthroscopy Pioneer, Inventor of "Tommy John" surgery, Founder of Kerlan-Jobe Orthopaedic Clinic, Clinical Professor of Orthopedics Keck School of Medicine, USC

Frank Jobe, M.D., co-founder of the famed Kerlan-Jobe Orthopaedic Clinic, inventor of Tommy John surgery, a pioneer in the use of arthroscopy and one of the most revered sports medicine surgeons ever.

On September 25, 1974, Jobe made sports medicine history when he performed the first reconstruction of the ulnar collateral ligament of the elbow (UCL) using a revolutionary procedure he had devised. It was performed on the, then Los Angeles major league pitcher named Tommy John. The procedure, commonly known as "Tommy John surgery" has become so prevalent an estimated one-third of all major league pitchers have undergone it.

Jobe also performed the first major reconstructive shoulder surgery on a big league player in 1990, which allowed Dodger star pitcher, Orel Hershiser, to continue his career.

For 40 years, Jobe served as the Los Angeles Dodger's team physician remaining on their medical staff through 2008. Dr. Jobe was also the orthopedic consultant for professional golf's PGA and Champions Tours for 26 years and named the emeritus physician for the PGA Tour.

Frank Jobe, notably, mentored Lewis Yocum, who was considered to be one of the best orthopedic surgeons in baseball when he died in May 2013.

Dr. Jobe's name has periodically been mentioned by sportswriters, fans, and players alike as worthy of a nomination for the National Baseball Hall of Fame. In

August 2012, an official campaign Web site to have Frank Jobe honored by the National Baseball Hall of Fame was launched.

Jobe was honored during Hall of Fame weekend on July 27, 2013, in Cooperstown, New York. Hall of Fame president Jeff Idelson said Jobe's work is a testament to the positive role of medicine in baseball's growth. Tommy John attended, praising Jobe by saying, "I think there should be a medical wing in the Hall of Fame, starting with him."

Frank Jobe was born in 1925 in Greensboro, North Carolina. After graduating from Collegedale Academy, he enlisted in the U.S. Army and went on to serve in World War II as a medical staff sergeant in the 101st Airborne Division.

He was captured and held for a short time as a prisoner of war during the Battle of the Bulge. He went on to earn the Bronze Star Medal, the Combat Medical Badge, and the Glider Badge.

Christopher Jobe, M.D., says of his father's military experience, "My dad was so impressed with the coolheaded doctors who had to care for patients with bullets flying everywhere. These were the moments that the idea of becoming a surgeon took hold."

Returning to the U.S., Dr. Jobe graduated from La Sierra University in Riverside, California, and obtained a medical degree from Loma Linda University. He was a general practitioner for three years, and then completed a residency in orthopedic surgery. In 1964 Jobe joined with Dr. Robert Kerlan to start the Southwestern Orthopaedic Medical Group in Los Angeles, which, in 1985, changed its name to the Kerlan-Jobe Orthopaedic Clinic.

Over the course of his career, Frank Jobe authored over 140 medical publications, wrote 30 book chapters, and edited seven books. He received three honorary doctorates, two from the United States and one from Japan.

Jobe also served as Clinical Professor in the Department of Orthopedics, Keck School of Medicine at the University of Southern California.

Dr. Christopher Jobe said of his father; "He was the most natural orthopedic surgeon I have ever watched. He wasn't one to start with theory and then come up with solution. He went directly from problem to solution; it was often the rest of us who sought out the theory. Everyone talks about the Tommy John surgery, but I think the greater intellectual feat was the surgery on Orel Hershiser. Dad worked out that extra stretch in the front of the shoulder that was responsible for problems in the back of the shoulder. He had a deeply intuitive understanding of biomechanics."

Neal ElAttrache, M.D.: "Frank was the most talented surgeon I have ever seen. When I joined the practice in 1990, he had begun to see that much of what had been done open probably could be done arthroscopically with less invasiveness.

So rather than be like his colleagues who stuck with open surgery, Frank embraced arthroscopy and encouraged me to embrace it. For a guy who made his reputation as an open shoulder and elbow surgeon to get up at meetings and say, 'arthroscopy is better' was really something."

James Bradley, M.D., "Frank Jobe was a humble, serene soul who could flat out operate better than anyone I've ever seen. He made even the most difficult cases look like a gentle waltz with those big size 9 hands. One day in 1988 (pre-MRIs) I asked Dr. Jobe how he knew that the ulnar collateral ligament in a certain MLB pitcher was incompetent. He said, 'sensitive fingers and thousands of physical exams,' and just smiled."

"This man touched the lives of so many surgeons and athletes with a soft encouraging word, kind smile and wink and by basically redefining the surgical approaches to the shoulder and elbow in the overhead athlete."

Norman A. Johanson

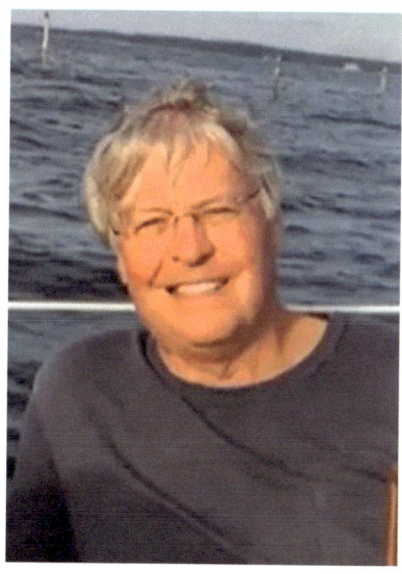

Born:	1950
Died:	2022
Years Active:	41
Location:	Philadelphia, Pennsylvania
Role(s):	Chief of Orthopedics Hahnemann University Hospital, Professor of Orthopedic Surgery Temple University School of Medicine, 2010 Sir John Charnley award winner from the Arthritis Foundation of Philadelphia, 2013 Distinguished Alumnus Award from HSS.

Norman A. Johanson, M.D., was the final chief of orthopedics at Hahnemann University Hospital, one of the oldest orthopedic academic institutions in the United States.

Johanson served in that position from 2000 until Hahnemann closed in 2019. Before that, he was a professor of orthopedic surgery and program director for 10 years at Temple University's School of Medicine, now the Lewis Katz School of Medicine.

Johanson started his practice at the Hospital for Special Surgery in New York City. Over the course of his career, Dr. Johanson published a multitude of medical papers and won several awards, including the 1978 T. Campbell Thompson Prize in orthopedic surgery from the Cornell University Medical College, now the Weill Medical College; the 2010 Sir John Charnley Award from the Arthritis Foundation in Philadelphia, and the 2013 Distinguished Alumnus Award from the Hospital for Special Surgery.

He was also active with the American Academy of Orthopaedic Surgeons, American Association of Hip and Knee Surgeons, Hip Society, and Philadelphia Orthopaedic Society.

Johanson was born June 16, 1950, in Greenwich, Connecticut to his parents, Wilbur Carl Johanson, an architect and artist, and Joy Segerstrom Johanson.

He ran track and field at Greenwich High School and at the 1968 state championship he set a high school record with a pole vault of 12 feet and 3 inches.

He continued his love of sports in college when he played football and studied biology and art history at Trinity College in Connecticut. When he graduated in 1972, he went on to Cornell University where he earned his medical degree in 1978.

One former colleague told *The Philadelphia Inquirer*, "When we are faced with a tough case or patient, we all ask ourselves: 'What would Norm do?' It is the highest compliment you could give a doctor."

Johanson believed it was his mission to help disadvantaged patients and even helped a woman organize a fundraiser to pay for her surgery.

Kiyoshi Kaneda

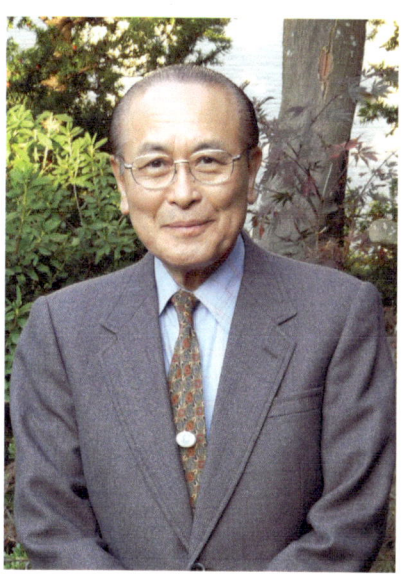

Born:	1936
Died:	2022
Years Active:	40+
Location:	Sapporo, Japan
Role(s):	Twice winner of the Leon Wiltse Award, winner of the Harrington Award by the Scoliosis Research Society, Inventor of the Kaneda Dual Rod system, Spine Surgery Pioneer

Kiyoshi Kaneda is one of the most consequential early pioneers of spine surgery, inventor of the Kaneda Dual Rod system, two time winner of the prestigious Wiltse Award for lifetime achievement and professor at the University of Hokkaido Medical School in Sapporo, Japan.

Well known to multiple generations of spine and neurosurgeons, in 2010, Professor Kaneda was awarded the Harrington Award by the Scoliosis Research Society at the spectacular Kyoto International Conference Center. In 2000 he won the Orthopaedic Research Society's Arthur B. Steindler Award.

Professor Kaneda's pivotal role in the history and development of Japanese and global spine surgery in advancing the care of patients with severe spinal deformities cannot be overstated. He is, among his other many accomplishments, the inventor of the Kaneda Dual Rod system.

In an interview with Orthopedics This Week, Professor Kaneda described his career.

"I am honored and privileged to receive the Leon Wiltse Award from the Society. Looking back, I would like to first recognize Harvard University's Professor John Hall. He extended an invitation to me to be a spine fellow with him at Harvard University in the 1970s."

"I didn't speak very much English at the time. But I went to Boston. After his lectures, Professor Hall would take the time to explain further his lectures. It was from Professor Hall that I began to learn anterior approaches for treating spinal deformities. I studied the Zielke, Dwyer, and Texas Scottish Rite approaches."

"In 1979 I returned to Japan and brought the anterior rod approach with me. But we had problems and difficulties. The single rod system couldn't handle the loads."

"Biomechanically, the single rod system had weaknesses. It only worked in two dimensions. So, we started testing a two rod design. With a dual rod, we were able to address spinal instability within a three dimension approach. The rods in the dual rod system were skinnier, but they provided more stability than a single rod. We have found that the dual rod system is effective for stabilization in many indications including deformities and vertebral fractures."

Professor's Kaneda served as professor and chairman of orthopedic surgery at Hokkaido University in Sapporo, Japan. Kaneda worked with Professor Manohar M. Panjabi, a Yale University expert on spinal trauma, and inspired his spine fellows to publish a significant body of biomechanical research.

Kaneda served as President of the International Society for the Study of the Lumbar Spine in 1996, an organization he'd been part of since 1981.

Kaneda was born in Fukushima Prefecture in Japan in 1936. He earned his medical degree at Hokkaido University School of Medicine in Sapporo, Japan, in 1962, completed an internship at Kyoto University Hospital and finished his orthopedic residency at Hokkaido University.

Kaneda was awarded a visiting clinical fellowship to learn scoliosis surgery and spinal instrumentation from Professor John E. Hall at Harvard Medical School and The Children's Hospital Medical Center in Boston. He was inspired by Hall's surgical techniques for anterior thoracolumbar instrumentation surgery known as "Dwyer instrumentation" and went on to further develop the techniques in his own practice.

After his fellowship, he returned to Hokkaido University and focused on scoliosis and spine surgeries. It was in early 1980s that he developed the Kaneda device and applied it treating thoracolumbar spinal injuries.

"Amazingly, even after making historic achievement, he read abstract book end to end and kept acquiring new knowledge throughout his life. He was a great surgeon, a great researcher, and a great teacher for us," wrote Mashairo Kanayma, of the International Society for the Study of the Lumbar Spine.

Professor Kaneda's legacy lives on in two principal forms – the patients he healed, the surgeons he trained and the many awards his colleagues gave him over the years.

2009 Whitecloud Award for Best Basic Science Paper. 16th Annual Meeting of the International Meeting of Advanced Spine Techniques (IMAST).

2002 Best Paper of the Society Award – Japanese Scoliosis Research Society.

2002 North American Spine Society (NASS) Award for Basic Science Spinal Research

2001 North American Spine Society (NASS) Award for Basic Science Spinal Research

2001 Moe Exhibit Award, Scoliosis Research Society

1998 Moe Exhibit Award, Scoliosis Research Society

1998 Japanese Spine Research Society Award for Basic Science

1992 Cervical Spine Research Society (CSRS) Basic Science Research Award

1991 North American Spine Society (NASS) Award for Spinal Research

1991 American Orthopaedic Association (AOA) Award for Orthopaedic Spinal Research

1991 Cervical Spine Research Society (CSRS) Residents Award for Cervical Spine Research

Michael A. Kelly

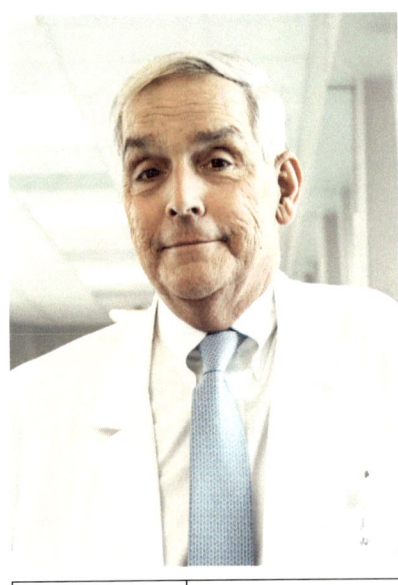

Born:	1952
Died:	2022
Years Active:	
Location:	Franklin Lakes, New Jersey
Role(s):	Pioneer in total knee arthroplasty, President of the American Knee Society, Founding Chair of orthopedic surgery at Hackensack Meridian School of Medicine, AAOS Lifetime Achievement Award Winner

Michael A. Kelly, M.D., founding chair of orthopedic surgery at Hackensack Meridian School of Medicine specialized in and taught hip and knee reconstructive surgery at Hackensack University Medical Center, where he was named chairman of orthopedic surgery and sports medicine in 2005.

A pioneer in total knee replacement, Kelly was also a founding member of Insall Scott Kelly Institute in New York and served as president of the American Knee Society, was head team physician for the New Jersey Nets basketball team.

Dr. Kelly received many awards during his career including Orthopedist of the Year by the New Jersey Arthritis Foundation and two Lifetime Achievement awards at the American Academy of Orthopedic Surgery.

Kelly attended Georgetown University Medical School and did his surgical internship and residency at St. Vincent's Hospital and Medical Center in New York City, and his orthopedic surgery training at Columbia Presbyterian Medical Center, also in New York City.

He then completed a knee surgery fellowship under Dr. John Insall, a pioneer in knee replacement surgery, at the Hospital for Special Surgery in New York City.

Kelly was born in Washington D.C. to Jacques Michael and Ann Muse Gillespie Kelly, but he grew up in Plainfield, New Jersey, before moving back to Washington, D.C. to attend Gonzaga College High

School. He received his bachelor's degree from the University of North Carolina at Chapel Hill.

"Michael was here at the School's beginnings—he played a critical role in establishing the Hackensack Meridian Health network. He was always a voice of reason; always expressing strong and constructive ideas as the school came together. He was an incredible mentor to our students and was bursting with pride when we placed a student in one of the most competitive orthopedics residencies in our first national match," said Jeffrey Boscamp, M.D., Interim Dean and Professor of Pediatrics at Hackensack Meridian School of Medicine.

Max E. Link

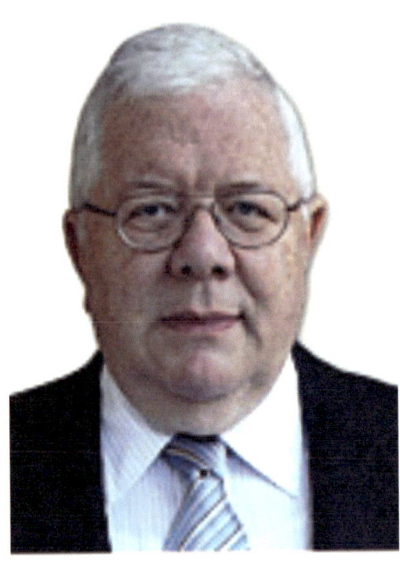

Max E. Link, Ph.D., was the former CEO of Corange, Ltd., the parent company of Boehringer Mannheim Therapeutics, Boehringer Mannheim Diagnostics and DePuy Orthopedics.

Dr. Link had also served as chairman and CEO of Centerpulse AG, a medical implant company later acquired by Zimmer Holdings, Inc.

He was actively involved as a director in numerous development-stage companies within the biopharmaceutical and medical device fields.

Dr. Link earned a Ph.D. in economics from University of St. Gallen (Switzerland).

Born:	1940
Died:	2014
Years Active:	
Location:	
Role(s):	Pioneering Orthopedic Manufacturing executive, CEO of Corange, owner of DePuy, CEO of Centerpulse (now part of Zimmer Biomet) and many other orthopedic companies.

Max Link was also the former chairman of the board of Sandoz Pharma, Ltd., CEO of Sandoz Pharma, and a member of the Executive Board of Sandoz, Ltd., Basel.

He also served as chairman of the board of directors of Alexion Pharmaceuticals, Inc., director, and the chairman of the board of directors at Celsion Corporation, as well as chairman of the board of directors at CytRx Corporation.

Leonard Bell, M.D., chairman and chief executive officer of Alexion, said, "Max's career was especially unique because he drove innovation on behalf of patients across so many areas of healthcare, including medical devices, pharmaceuticals—and biotechnology."

"As Chairman, he was a key guide in our transition from a development-stage company to our current multinational commercial platform."

"Max was committed to, and excited by, innovation. Likewise, he was a strong believer in the power of entrepreneurship and saw this as a vital engine for meeting patients' needs."

Dr. Link served as Amedica Corporation's chairman of the board of directors from October 2003 until his retirement in August 2014.

Gregg Honigblum, managing director at Westlake Securities noted, "Max was one of the most intelligent and respected icons in the healthcare field. His integrity was his greatest attribute."

John Thomas Makley

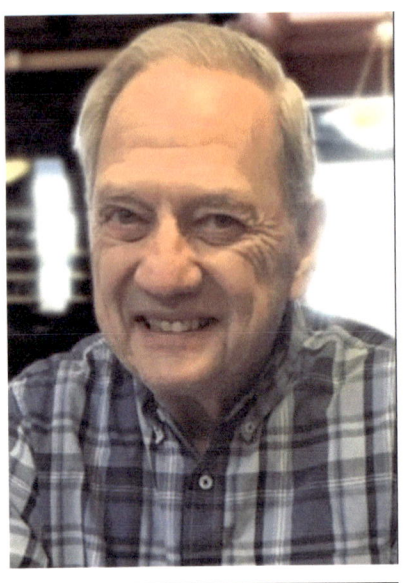

Born:	1936
Died:	2020
Years Active:	50+
Location:	Cleveland, Ohio
Role(s):	Professor of Medicine, Case Western Reserve Medical School and University Hospitals, long-time Musculoskeletal Transplant Foundation board member, founding member Musculoskeletal Tumor Society

John Thomas Makley, M.D. was a titan of the global orthopedic community. A renowned orthopedic surgeon, Dr. Makley was also professor of medicine at Case Western Reserve University Medical School and University Hospitals in Cleveland and a long-time member of the Medical Board of Trustees at the Musculoskeletal Tissue Foundation.

Makley specialized in oncology and musculoskeletal tumors and had a national influence on these fields over the course of his half a century long career.

He was an innovator in the national treatment of bone and soft-tissue tumors as well as bone banking.

Born in southern Ohio as the youngest of five siblings, Makley followed in the footsteps of his older brother, Tod, an ophthalmologist, and dreamed of becoming a doctor from a young age. After graduating from University of Dayton in 1957, he enrolled in the University of Cincinnati Medical School.

In 1961, Makley graduated from University of Cincinnati Medical School and interned at University Hospital. Here, Makley worked under the mentorship of Charles Herndon, M.D., who would be a lifelong mentor. Makley chose to pursue specialties in both orthopedic surgery and oncology. He then procured a year-long fellowship residency at the University of Florida in Gainesville in 1968.

In 1969, Makley began a position in Cleveland's Orthopaedics Department at

University Hospitals. He embarked upon a remarkable 50-year career as a surgeon and researcher.

Makley and his research partners explored a range of research topics and issues regarding cancer diagnosis and treatment, musculoskeletal tumors and infectious disease. Makley and his colleagues Charles Hubay, M.D., and Arnold Powell, M.D., Ph.D., developed a ground-breaking cancer screening test that requires only a small blood sample.

Makley and his mentor John Carter, M.D., published over 50 orthopedic journal articles through the 70s, 80s, 90s and early 2000s. Makley was a founding member of the Musculoskeletal Tumor Society in 1977. The group focused on policy-making with the needs of patients and their orthopaedic oncologists in mind. The Society now has over 150 members worldwide and now sponsors fellowships.

In 1991, Makley received a "Distinguished Alumni Award" at his Alma Mater, the University of Dayton. In 2000, Makley retired from University Hospitals. He and his colleagues received the Carter-Makley-Theros lectureship in Musculoskeletal Pathology a few years later.

Finally, Dr. Makley made further contributions as a physician when he returned to a part-time position at the Cleveland Veteran Affairs Medical Center's Orthopaedic Surgery unit as an orthopedic oncologist in the late 2000s. There, Dr. Makley staffed a large number of out-patient consults and offered non-operative care. He retired from the VAMC in 2015.

Martha Anderson, EVP, Donor Services of MTF Biologics said, of Dr. Makley, " "Dr. Makley was a long-time member of the Medical Board of Trustees of MTF Biologics (also known as the Musculoskeletal Transplant Foundation) and MTF's Board of Directors. His commitment to and compassion for his patients were only matched by his surgical expertise, commitment to education and sense of humor. The Board of Directors and staff of MTF Biologics mourn his loss and appreciate his contributions to advancing the science of orthopaedic oncology and transplantation."

Thomas Mallory

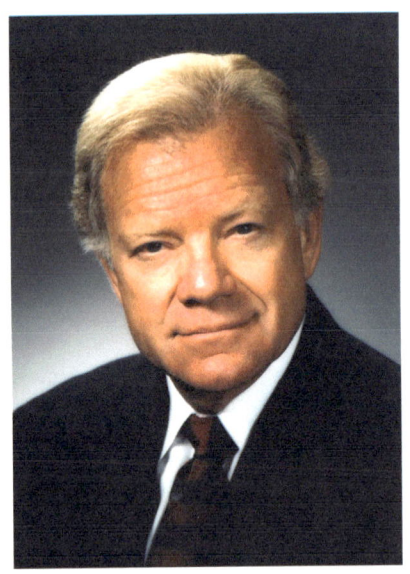

Born:	1939
Died:	2019
Years Active:	
Location:	Columbus, Ohio
Role(s):	Performed 1st hip replacement surgery in the United States, inventor of the Mallory Head Total Hip System, founder and 1st Chairman of the Department of Orthopedics at Ohio State University.

Thomas Mallory, M.D., of Loudonville, Ohio, was one of the essential pioneers in the field of orthopedic surgery.

Dr. Mallory performed the first U.S. total hip replacement surgery in Columbus, Ohio, in 1971. Dr. Mallory was also responsible for co-creating the innovative Mallory Head Total Hip System, a comprehensive hip prosthetic technology that is now used internationally. He also created a significant body of professional accomplishments and research which moved the field of orthopedic surgery forward on multiple levels.

Dr. Mallory was born on January 10, 1939, in Hillsboro, Ohio. He completed his bachelor's degree at Miami University in Oxford, Ohio, where he lettered in varsity football during each of those four years.

Dr. Mallory entered medical school at the Ohio State University College of Medicine in 1961. Dr. Mallory completed both his medical training and orthopedic residency at Ohio State. In addition, Dr. Mallory completed a research fellowship at Tufts University. He was also a hip surgery fellow at Harvard Medical School. He would go on to engage in several decades of clinical practice, research, teaching, training, and study.

Between 1965 and 1974, Mallory served in the 2291st Medical Corps as a Reserve Officer. In 1971, Dr. Mallory performed the first full hip replacement in the United States at the Ohio State University Hospital.

The following year, Dr. Mallory founded Joint Implants Surgeons (JIS), a practice specializing in total hip and total knee replacement where he actively practiced medicine for 30 years.

Dr. Mallory had a vision for an efficient and evidence-based surgical practice. Mallory's vision was for "an orthopaedic surgery center that would embody this commitment by continually developing methodologies that allowed for ever-greater efficiencies in both the operating room and post-operative care." He employed a patient-centered, research-driven team approach to clinical care that was unique in the time he began practicing. Dr. Mallory's vision for JIS eventually gave life to New Albany Surgical Hospital, a surgery center specializing in orthopedic care.

In addition to writing and contributing to hundreds of publications throughout the course of his clinical career, Dr. Mallory was fascinated with biomedical engineering and co-created a hip prosthesis. Along with Ohio State University professorial colleague Dr. William C. Head, he designed the Mallory-Head Hip Implant System. Marketed by Biomet in 1984, the cementless prosthesis became rapidly employed worldwide as a technology that leaves hip replacement patients with less chronic pain.

Dr. Mallory founded the Department of Orthopaedics at Ohio State University College of Medicine. He filled the role of initial chair and was later Emeritus Chairman of this department. During his term as active Chairman, he was at the helm of efforts to procure the present Ohio State University Wexner Medical Center East.

In 2007, Dr. Mallory published a professional memoir, *The Man Behind the Mask*, in which he. described introducing full hip replacement surgery policies and his innovative advocacy for modularity techniques which allowed surgeons to customize prostheses to patient joints during surgery.

In 2001, Dr. Mallory was diagnosed with Parkinson's disease. He continued to apply his sharp intellect and critical thinking skills to the exploration of his illness. After empirical observation of his improvement through the benefits of diet and exercise, Mallory developed a new exercise treatment for delaying the Parkinson's symptom progression. This regimen, called "Delay the Disease," is now utilized at OhioHealth and various international treatment centers.

Adolph Lombardi, Jr., M.D. described Dr. Mallory as a charismatic man and an enthusiastic lifelong learner. He recalled that Dr. Mallory recommended that those in the field "read one new article every day" and "always seek to expand your knowledge base. Always seek to be better than you are today."

Dr. Lombardi described meeting Mallory at an American Academy of Orthopaedic Surgeons continuing education conference in 1983, stating he was "in awe of this vibrant, energetic, captivating, and charismatic professor.

"I lived 15 minutes away, he lived an hour and a half away, and he was there 20 minutes before everyone else arrived. At 4:45 AM, he was there, ready to go, charged up. Do you think he was a lounge lizard?"

"He never sat in the lounge. He never drank coffee between cases. He was always in the operating room, he was always ready to go, he was always motivating and inspiring. We could mop the floors, we could move the patient, we could change the bed, because we had the ticket. We had a license to practice medicine, we had a license to do the surgery, and if we were ready to go, the team was moving forward. This is what he taught us from day one."

Keith Berend, M.D., another of Dr. Mallory's esteemed colleagues at JIS said of Dr. Mallory:

"When I joined Joint Implant Surgeons JIS in 2002, Dr. Mallory had retired from operating. However, his mentorship and guidance was invaluable early in my career and continues to be so. He taught me the three most important pillars of a successful practice. These were education and training the future surgeons, research, and patient care. These three pillars of practice continue to be the foundation by which JIS orthopedics remain successful in my own practice I'm able to remain relevant. It is with sincere gratitude that I had the honor to have worked with Dr. Mallory and have him mentor me early in my career."

Henry J. Mankin

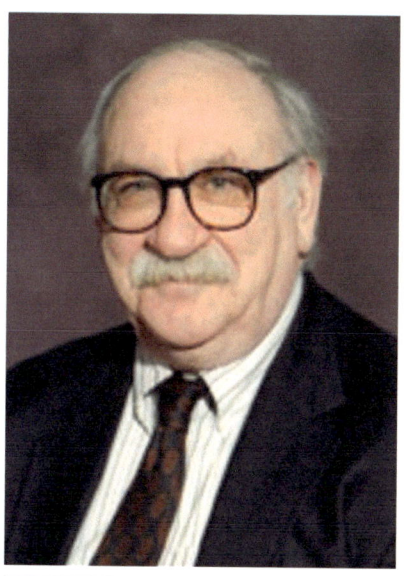

Born:	1928
Died:	2018
Years Active:	50+
Location:	Boston, Massachusetts
Role(s):	Chief of Orthopedics at Mass General, Harvard Medical School, Cleveland Clinic, Hospital for Joint Disease and Mount Sinai Medical Center, Author of essential textbooks in Orthopedic Surgery.

There is a special place in the pantheon of orthopedic surgeons for Henry J. Mankin, M.D., a world-renown musculoskeletal surgeon, educator, scientist and mentor whose orthopedic career spanned over 50 years.

A native of Pittsburgh, Henry Mankin attended the University of Pittsburgh for both his undergraduate and medical degrees. Dr. Mankin remembered, "Our class had 100 people, only five of whom were women; compare that with this year's class at Harvard, which has 54% women."

During his internal medicine internship at the University of Chicago, Henry Mankin was called upon to work as a Naval physician in Nevada. He said, "I got my introduction to orthopedics courtesy of some of the military folks around me who got into fights and broke one another's limbs."

In 1957 Dr. Mankin entered the residency program at The Hospital for Joint Diseases in New York City (later NYU Langone Orthopedic Hospital), after which time he spent six years at the University of Pittsburgh.

In 1966 he returned to the Hospital for Joint Diseases as chief of service and professor at Mt. Sinai.

Dr. Mankin would spend the next 40 years of his career as the chief of orthopedics at the Massachusetts General Hospital and at Harvard Medical School.

Freddie Fu, M.D. said of his dear friend

and colleague, "A legend in orthopaedics, Dr Mankin's contribution to education, research and patient care in our field around the world is tremendous and forever lasting. His iconic, down to earth, and funny demeanor made him so very special!"

The winner of 2004 Diversity Award from the American Academy of Orthopaedic Surgeons, Dr. Mankin was ahead of his time.

Constance Chu, M.D. said of her friend and mentor, "Henry Mankin was an inspirational leader who embraced diversity in orthopedic surgery long before it was fashionable. I met him in an elevator at the Mass General in 1991."

"After hearing that I had graduated from West Point and was interested in orthopedics, he ushered me out at Gray 6 where he introduced me to the large team waiting for him and then exuberantly announced, 'She is going to be an orthopedic surgeon.' Shortly thereafter, he shared with me his reverence for articular cartilage and challenged me to figure out how to heal cartilage and prevent osteoarthritis. He was an incredible figure who inspired and shaped the careers of countless orthopedic surgeons, who opened the door for women and minorities, and who devoted himself to everything about orthopedics."

Dr. Mankin established a computerized system for tumors that includes all of the tumor patients he treated since 1972. He completed two volumes of the pathology and physiology of orthopedic disease. Dr. Mankin said, "I believe the books are particularly useful for residents, fellows, and people in clinical science. In composing these books I have held in mind that we need to determine the best way to operate on patients and the simplest way to treat fractures. We must consider disease states, what they mean, and what we can understand from them about bones, soft tissue, and joints."

Said Mark C. Gebhardt, M.D., "Whether you knew him or not, you have been influenced by his teachings. At every residency graduation he would start with, 'Classes come, and classes go...' and then would talk about teaching as the highest profession; because your challenge as a teacher is for your students to go on and do better and more wonderful things than you could ever imagine as their teacher. And that will remain his ageless legacy."

Bruno Melzi

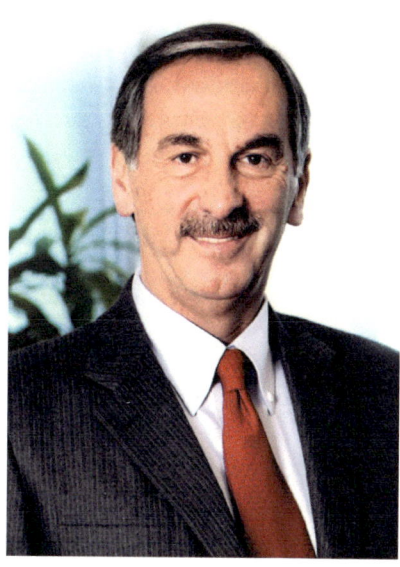

Born:	1948
Died:	2020
Years Active:	47
Location:	Milan, Italy
Role(s):	Former President of Zimmer Europe, former Managing Director of Johnson & Johnson's orthopedic business in Italy and a pioneer in building orthopedics throughout Europe.

Dr. Bruno Melzi was President of Zimmer, International, member of LimaCorporate board of directors and president of the Brunenghi di Castelleone Foundation, among many other roles and responsibilities.

Dr. Melzi began his orthopedic career in 1973 with Johnson & Johnson where he eventually became the managing director for all of Italy. In 1990, he joined Zimmer as managing director for Italy and 10 years after that, became president of Zimmer International.

Dr. Melzi also held managerial positions with Eucomed, played a key role in Zimmer's integration of Centerpulse and was a member of LimaCorporate's board of directors.

Dr. Melzi held a law degree from University of Pavia.

Of all Dr. Melzi's accomplishments, and there are very many, his work in his beloved hometown of Castelleone, which is located just south of Milan, Italy, gave him the most joy. The foundation to which he dedicated himself to operates a 124-bed nursing home for residents of the immediate area.

In 2015 Dr. Melzi said this about joining the Brunenghi foundation: "I love my country [...] and I have always had the desire to do something for my fellow citizens—to put my professional experience available to my community. A positive ambition that I always had even when I lived far away. So, when I was offered the assignment, it seemed almost natural to accept, it was the opportunity I had been waiting for, for a long time, almost without knowing it."

Milan's vicar general Fr Massimo Calvi wrote a public note in honor and remembrance of Dr. Melzi saying: "I like to remember the active and proactive participation in our meetings, constantly animated in the common reflections by the desire for concreteness and the desire to encourage ever greater collaboration between the various Foundations. I express my deepest condolences and assure you of a fraternal and grateful remembrance in prayer for him and his family members."

A few months before he fell ill, Bruno Melzi had started his second term as president of the Brunenghi Foundation. And soon after that, Dr. Melzi had been confirmed as a representative of the Diocese of Cremona on the Board of Directors of the Foundation that manages the Castelleone rsa.

According to those who knew Dr. Melzi best, he was blessed with an extroverted and warm, sympathetic personality. He was famous for being able to relate and converse with all people, on an amazingly wide range of subjects whether it was his beloved Milan soccer teams or the latest in orthopedic medicine and corporate work to politics or the economy. His friends say that he had the great ability to put anyone at ease and could switch from the Castellan dialect to Italian to English and more.

Ray Elliott, former chief executive officer at Zimmer Corporation said, of Dr. Melzi, "I knew Bruno for thirty years, first as a tough competitor and then as a friend and partner at Zimmer but always close, always honorable. I can still see us now ... laughing together so many times."

"Bruno, should we ever move the head office to Roma?" The response ... 'Roma is a beautiful, romantic city but my bella would divorce me, my son disown me, the employees hate me, my beloved farm gone ... you would find me alone, driving in THAT traffic forced to have my pasta WITH red sauce !!!!!'"

"I have been convinced for the longest time that our annual sales goals for Bruno and the European team were consistently lost somewhere between the risotto and the grappa."

"Under that knowing smile, effortless charm and smooth conversation was a warmth a whole room could feel ... what they may not have known is that it came from the fire of a relentless competitor."

John Cresser-Brown recalls, "Bruno Melzi was like a business father to many of us that worked in his organisation. He inspired success and loyalty, and always had time to guide and direct his team with unwavering leadership."

Audrey Beckman, former senior vice president, Strategic Quality Initiatives, Zimmer Biomet said, "Bruno was a leader who shared stories, all with points to understand and learn from, yet he could lighten a serious atmosphere with just one comment. He knew the diverse European orthopaedic market intimately and worked tirelessly to shape it, with a keen sense of what was needed to improve patient care."

Michael Humphris, Vice President Europe, recalls, "I had the privilege of working alongside Mr. Melzi for 20 years. Bruno was an intensely loyal man, very proud of his European team, a man of natural charisma and leadership, we all have reason to thank him for the successes he shared with us, and for leading us through a period of enormous change in the company and the industry."

Sheryl Conley, former group president, Americas, Global Marketing, and chief marketing officer, Zimmer Biomet said, "Bruno was passionate about business, his family and his village. Often, he opened up his home to his friends and colleagues and I had a chance to see what he loved about Castelleone."

"I can't count how many times we'd walk through the streets and people would come up to him and ask his advice about politics or other matters. As we walked, he would humbly and proudly show me the historical buildings and cultural landmarks whose restoration he had personally invested."

"Bruno had the ability to truly make people welcome and he also was a leader who had the ability to assess business issues and drive a team to a conclusion diplomatically and with his great sense of humor. 'Sheryl', he often said to me, 'business is very serious, but there is also the life.' I will be forever grateful for having Bruno as a mentor, colleague and especially a friend."

Antony Massarella, former vice president, North Europe, Zimmer Biomet said, "It was a great honour for me to be part of Dr. Melzi's management team for 15 years. During that time, he led us through some very exciting and challenging events including several acquisitions, periods of economic turbulence, regulatory upheaval and technological disruption. Throughout all of that his intense focus on protecting and growing our business retained a strong emphasis on personal accountability. He was without question a highly demanding manager to work for, but his managerial logic was consistent and fair with a degree of tolerance. I recall his staff meetings in Milan with warmth because, while they could be tough and often highly stressful, they were not without elements of fun given his ever-present and highly idiosyncratic brand of humour. Dr. Melzi was, without question, an inspirational and charismatic leader, I learned a great deal from him."

Dane A. Miller

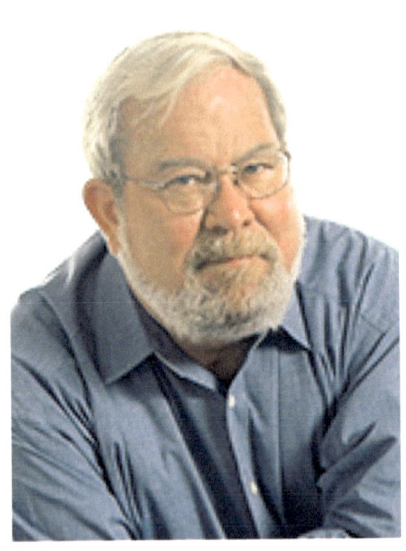

Born:	1946
Died:	2015
Years Active:	40+
Location:	Warsaw, Indiana
Role(s):	Co-founder of Biomet, one of the largest orthopedic companies in the world, essential entrepreneur and executive in modern orthopedic history, mentor and partner to two generations of orthopedic executives and surgeons.

Dane A. Miller, Ph.D., was the co-founder and CEO of Biomet, Inc. and is one of the most essential entrepreneurs and executives in orthopedic manufacturing, teaching, product development and, indeed, the entire process of translating ideas into clinically relevant products and techniques.

As the Jeff Binder, at the time CEO of Biomet, said, "It is impossible in one short statement to give justice to his impact on our company, on our industry, and on the communities where we operate—especially Warsaw and Winona Lake, Indiana. It is also impossible to describe adequately Dane's impact on the lives of our Team Members and on the members of the orthopaedic community with whom he worked and developed friendships over many years."

Dane was born in Bellefontaine, Ohio. He and the former Mary Louise Schilke met as teens in Springfield, Ohio, at a swim club. They were married on February 19, 1966.

In the beginning the young couple moved every six weeks between Dayton, Ohio, where Miller worked, and Flint, Michigan, so he could attend General Motors Institute (now Kettering University). He earned a master's degree and, later, a Ph.D. in bio-medical engineering from the University of Cincinnati.

With those credentials, the couple began his professional career at the Frigidaire Division, GMC in Dayton, Ohio, from

1964 to 1969, working as a cooperative engineering student. From 1972 to 1975 he was employed as the director of biomedical engineering at Zimmer. His responsibilities included engineering, prototype design and fabrication, as well as basic research support for all new product development programs. He was also responsible for coordinating and developing a custom and special product group, including marketing, sales, and manufacturing of custom products.

From 1975 to 1977, he was Director of Biomedical Engineering for Cutter Biomedical, a division of Cutter Laboratories, Inc.

Dane, Ferguson, Niles Noblitt and Ray Harroff founded Biomet, Inc. in 1977. Biomet—Bio for Body, met for metallurgical implants.

When Dane, Niles and Ray started Biomet in a converted barn in Warsaw, Indiana, they and their respective families had to financially scale back and live frugally.

The group had just $725, 000 of their own money, including a $500, 000 loan from the Small Business Administration. They posted a $63, 000 net loss the first year.

The wives took turns baby-sitting so they could go to the office and sweep the floors, type out invoices or answer phones. The men scrubbed toilets, picked up garbage, took orders and shipped product.

Garry England, the company's 41st employee said in a published interview, "I remember Dane doing wiring, office construction, sweeping, shoveling snow. It was a 'get-it-done' attitude that was very motivational to us (employees). In those days, you knew everybody who worked here by their first name; you knew their spouses' names and half their kids' names."

The financial risk was big, and the families put it all on the line. Dane and Mary Louise had personal guarantees of over $1 million dollars in debt and at the time had a net worth of $100, 000.

Instead of intimidating him, the prospect of failure inspired Dane. "Webster's dictionary really should carry his picture next to 'tenacity' because Dane never gives up, " Ferguson said in a published interview. "I mean he never gives up. It doesn't matter how bad things get." As a devout Presbyterian, Dane said he's not alone. "I rely on my spiritual underpinnings to keep me upright and moving forward."

"If we tried and failed, we were still young enough to pick ourselves up and try again, " Dane told students at the Kelley School of Business as part of the Distinguished Entrepreneur-in-Residence Series. "You don't want to look back and say, 'I wish I'd tried.' The risk of failure for start-up companies is very high. So? You start over again."

One of the goals of the new company was to take suggestions from orthopedic surgeons and come out with improved implants faster than their big competitors.

Right from the start, the priorities were: solid engineering, customer responsiveness, superior clinical results and top-notch quality.

Dane said the company's culture was about taking a hands-on approach to their business. "Our employees get it done. There is no job at Biomet that isn't everyone's job. It's our company. As we grow larger, we don't want to drift into a habit of acting as if we're all managers, not employees or shareholders."

By early 1979 most of their seed money was gone. But the group was able to obtain $500,000 in equity from a venture capital investor and kept Biomet afloat until the first profitable year, 1980.

By 1980, Biomet earned $1.1 million in net sales. The company went public in 1981, had Wall Street's attention by 1983, and in 1987, with $96.7 million in net sales, was deemed a "hot growth company." In 1984, Dane predicted Biomet would be a billion dollar company by 2000.

"They all thought I was nuts, " said Dane. "How could anyone imagine by the year 2000 we'd be doing a billion dollars? And, in fact, in the fiscal year 2000, we reached a billion dollars."

There were some technology hiccups.

In 1983, came the Dermizip, which was lauded as the "sizzle" that sold the August 1983 public offering of 3 million shares. This product was supposed to catapult Biomet into the surgical wound closure market. So, of course, Dane had the new "attachment apparatus" used on his own arm.

But, it didn't hold. Not one to quit, Dane flew to O'Hare Airport to meet John Sheehan, M.D., the surgeon who had designed the product. There, in the hallway, Dane had the original product replaced and flew off to Europe. After ten days and no healing, he had the Dermzip removed in Sweden.

Dermizip never formally went to market and in-house it became known as "Dermiscar." Dane was the only person to have it implanted.

Dane didn't just use his own devices on himself, his grandmother, Grace Shumaker, was the first recipient of a Biomet-made artificial hip.

Where Dane ended and Biomet began was essentially a non-existent boundary. Customers who needed to call him could reach Dane Miller at home. Dane was, perhaps, the only major orthopedic company CEO who handed out his home and cell phone numbers to customers. His home phone number was listed in the Warsaw, Indiana, phone book. He also, famously, answered his own phone in the office."

He ate in the Biomet cafeteria where he stood in line, getting a tray and sitting with a new group of employees every week. On business trips, Dane visited hospitals, scrubbed up, put on the surgical gown and watched surgeries. With a doctorate in biomedical engineering, Dane was at home with surgeons, his employees, his products, and his company.

And he was the fellow who has mentored hundreds of senior marketing and manufacturing managers in the nuts, bolts, screws and stems of this industry.

Merrill Ritter, M.D., a Mooresville, Indiana, orthopedic surgeon, said, "Dane is just a regular guy, but he is a very brilliant guy. He doesn't push his brightness; it just flows out of him."

Todd Albert, M.D., Surgeon in Chief and Medical Director at Hospital for Special Surgery in New York said Dane was an "amazing man—innovative, brilliant yet extremely down to earth.

Dane built Biomet into a company with 6, 000 worldwide employees under his watch.

Dane Miller was also director of Kosciusko Community Hospital, a member of the President's Council for Grace College and Seminary, a board member of the Kosciusko Leadership Academy and a board member of the University of Chicago Hospitals and Health System.

Maurice Edmond Muller

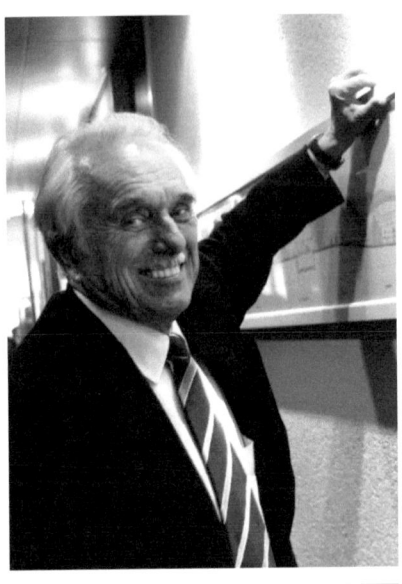

Maurice Edmond Müller's imagination and invisible hand guides every orthopedic surgeon performing surgery today.

His work described below may have made him the most influential surgeon of the 20th century.

The international organization of orthopedic surgeons (SICOT) recognized Dr. Müller's unique talents and contributions to science by naming him "The Orthopedic Surgeon of the Century" a few years ago.

Dr. Müller's influence on orthopedics cannot be overstated.

A small list of Dr. Müller's accomplishments includes;

- Invented the "Straight Stem" hip and instrumentation in 1977 that is still sold by Zimmer today and is inside over 1 million patients
- Performed over 20, 000 surgeries (4, 000 hip replacements)
- Founding Father of AO with four fellow Swiss surgeons
- Wrote 250 scientific papers
- Received 14 honorary degrees from universities around the world
- Developed the most comprehensive system of classification (The Müller AO Classification of Fractures in Long Bones) in 1990 for fractures and orthopedic surgery outcomes, which became the "universal language for orthopedic surgeons."

Born:	1918
Died:	2009
Years Active:	50+
Location:	Switzerland
Role(s):	Founding member of the AO Foundation, invented "Straight Stem" hip and instrumentation, wrote 250 published papers, received 14 honorary degrees, developed the The Müller AO Classification of Fractures in Long Bones

- Lead author of the 409-page "Manuel der Osteosynthese: AO-Technik" published in 1977

Maurice Edmond Müller was born in the last year of the Great War, 1918, in a village that sat on the border of the German and French speaking Swiss areas, Biel, Switzerland. He received his medical degree in 1946 and described his moment of epiphany in an undated interview with Maitrise Orthopedique.

"From the age of eight, my only ambition was to become a surgeon. I should mention that my father had been a surgeon in the States but had to give up his career to live in Switzerland, because his wife did not want to move to the USA."

"At the age of 20, after some psychometric tests, my choice of profession was approved by the experts. They told me that their tests had identified a three-dimensional gift, which could be used to advantage in orthopaedic surgery. After my state medical examinations in 1944 I worked as a locum GP for three weeks."

"Two patients made a particular impression on me. The gait of the first was normal. He told me he had fractured his femur during the war between Finland and Russia in 1940 and that a German military surgeon named Küntscher had operated on him at the front and inserted a long nail."

"Less than two weeks later he was walking comfortably with just one stick. At that time, this was amazing. He had only come in to find out where he should go to have his nail removed."

"The other patient was having trouble walking with a stick. When I suggested that he must be in great pain he replied: 'No, I am extremely well. Two years ago, I had a Leveuf hip arthroplasty. Before that I had been in excruciating pain both day and night; my hip had seized in a very poor position. It's true that my hip is now unstable, and I can't walk without a stick, but at least I can move it and it doesn't hurt. This operation has changed my life.'"

"Two weeks later I had decided to devote my surgical career firstly to fracture fixation and secondly to hip surgery. I was convinced that one of these fields would eventually revolutionize orthopaedic surgery. During the next 15 years, they became the most important aspects of orthopaedics, and my workload increased accordingly."

After graduating in 1946 from medical school in Lausanne, Dr. Müller chose, as his first posting, to volunteer for medical service in Ethiopia which helped to round out his medical education.

In 1950 Dr. Müller visited Robert Danis in Brussels, Belgium. Danis had achieved stable osteosynthesis through plates with compression devices. His methods allowed the patient immediate mobilization of the injured extremities and prevented the stiffness and disability, which were seen with traditional methods.

The techniques he witnessed with Danis formed the basis of the future AO technologies which Dr. Müller would help to systemize.

Word of his astounding technique in the operating room led a group of friends to coalesce around Maurice, men who would go on to form the Die Arbeitgemeinschaft für Osteosynthesefragen or AO Foundation – which, notably, was founded in Biel, Switzerland, Dr. Müller's birthplace.

Probably one of Dr. Müller's greatest accomplishments was trick was his collaboration with instrument maker Robert Mathys, a full range of AO implants within two short years.

To ensure a continuous flow of money for AO activities, Dr. Müller donated all of his intellectual property rights for the good of the AO. He showed his heart for others again in 1967 when he founded the M E Müller Foundation and also endowed chairs of orthopedic surgery in several countries. The museum in Bern dedicated to the famous Swiss born painter, the Paul Klee Zentrum, was only made possible thanks to the generosity of Maurice and his late wife Marti.

His name will live on in the Müller AO Classification of Fractures in Long Bones, which was released in 1990 and has become a worldwide standard.

Bruce D. Browner, M.D., FACS, called Dr. Müller the architect of modern fracture surgery as he presented Dr. Müller for an Honorary Fellowship in the American College of Surgeons (ACS).

Prior to Müller fractures had been treated since the mid-1800s with plaster and traction.

Added Browner, "In 1958, the dream of organizing an Association of Internal Fixation was realized, with the formation of the Die Arbeitgemeinschaft für Osteosynthesefragen or AO, which is roughly translated into the Association for the Study of Internal Fixation (ASIF)."

Jesse Jupiter, M.D., former Chair of AAOS' International Committee and Chief of the Hand and Upper Extremity Service in the Department of Orthopaedic Surgery at Massachusetts General Hospital said of Müller:

"While a world-class hip surgeon, Dr. Müller's real impact on patients around the world was his evolution, with several other Swiss surgeons, to develop the AO which revolutionized not only the treatment of fractures but also traumatic injuries as a whole."

"He was instrumental in developing surgical education with hands-on training, decades in advance of others, and clinical and basic research into traumatic injuries to the musculoskeletal system which has culminated in a world renown[ed] research center."

"Last but not least, in the era of evidence-based medicine, [Dr. Müller] was really among the first to establish documentation as the foundation of understanding the outcomes of the efforts of his colleagues in the AO."

"I really believe that his impact worldwide far eclipses Charnley or just about any other orthopaedic surgeon in the 20th century regarding the improvement in the treatment of musculoskeletal injuries and reconstruction to become the standard of care for most countries in the world."

Dr. h.c. mult. Hansjörg Wyss, former Executive Chairman of Synthes said of Müller:

"Maurice Müller's legacy lives on in the millions of patients who have been treated according to the AO principals he was central in creating."

"He was one of the true icons of modern orthopedics, having made a profound and lasting impact on fracture treatment, total joint replacement, and corrective and reconstructive surgery."

Biomet Founder Dane Miller, Ph.D. said, "Prof. Maurice Müller was a true pioneer in total joint replacement and trauma. His scientific approach to clinical and data collection set a standard never before achieved by a clinician."

Arthur M. Pappas

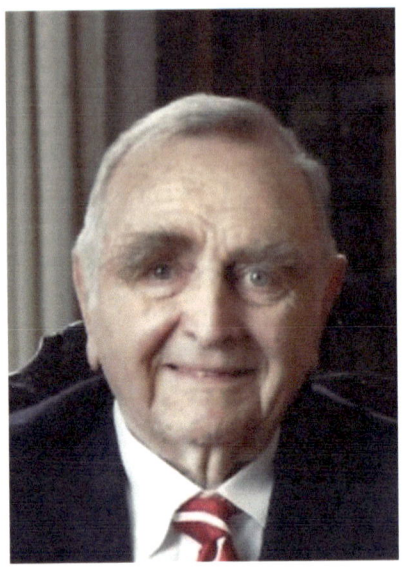

Born:	1932
Died:	2016
Years Active:	30+
Location:	Boston, Massachusetts
Role(s):	1st chairman of the Department of Orthopedics at the University of Massachusetts Medical School, Boston Red Sox team doctor, President of the Association of Professional Baseball Physicians.

Arthur M. Pappas, M.D. was a pioneering orthopedic and sports medicine physician. He was the first chairman of the Department of Orthopedics at the University of Massachusetts Medical School and, for 25 years, the Boston Red Sox's team physician and medical director.

Dr. Pappas was born and raised in Auburn, Massachusetts; he and his wife lived in the house in which Dr. Pappas was born.

Dr. Pappas chaired the boards of directors at Fairlawn Rehabilitation Hospital and the Massachusetts Hospital School for handicapped children and worked with Eunice Kennedy Shriver to establish the Special Olympics in Massachusetts.

Dr. Pappas graduated from Harvard College and attending medical school at the University of Rochester. He then spent two years in the U.S. Navy as a researcher at the National Naval Medical Center in Bethesda, Maryland.

Dr. Pappas played football at Harvard. Later, Dr. Pappas became the medical director for the Boston Red Sox in 1978 and stayed for over 25 years.

He served as president of the Association of Professional Baseball Physicians, was a member of the Sports Medicine Committee for the American Academy of Pediatrics, and also president of the Massachusetts Amateur Sports Foundation.

In 2011, Dr. Pappas, who was the chairman emeritus of the department of orthopedics and physical rehabilitation at UMass Memorial Medical Center, received the Massachusetts Medical Society's Lifetime Achievement Award.

Dr. Pappas received many honors, including the Massachusetts Medical Society Lifetime Achievement Award, the Massachusetts Hospital School's Edward H. Bradford Lifetime Achievement Award for Program Development for Handicapped Children, and the Physician Achievement Award from the Arthritis Foundation.

In 2012, a ribbon was cut on the $4.3 million Dr. Arthur Pappas and Dr. Martha Pappas Recreation Complex on Pakachoag Hill; the couple donated $1 million toward the park's construction, which includes baseball and soccer fields, a playground, and a performance stage.

The Pappas family also donated $763,000 to increase the size of the new high school's gymnasium. They established the Auburn Foundation through the Greater Worcester Community Foundation, which has awarded grants to Auburn-based nonprofit organizations since 2004.

Eric Dickson, M.D., president and CEO of UMass Memorial Health Care said about Dr. Pappas, "I think Art's passion was a belief that each day he could help improve the quality of life for the patients coming to see him. Dr. Pappas worked a great deal with handicapped children. He was one of the finest doctors in the country."

Charles Ray

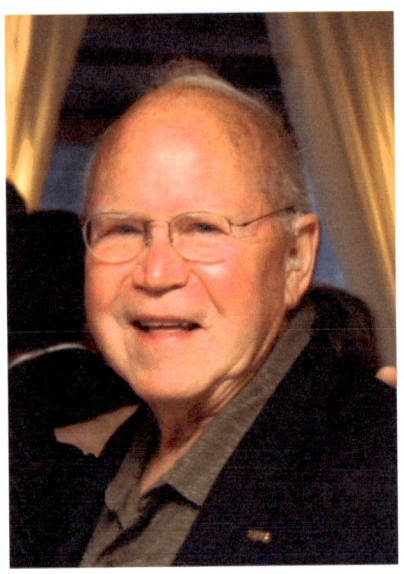

Born:	1927
Died:	2011
Years Active:	50+
Location:	Baltimore, MD
Role(s):	Co-founder North American Spine Society and other surgeon societies, Disc Arthroplasty pioneer, holder of 53 U.S. patents, 100+ foreign patents, author of more than 365 journal articles.

Charles Ray, M.D., played a larger-than-life role in shaping the surgical treatment of debilitating back pain, Dr. Ray, whose long list of inventions, patents, students and surgical techniques only begins to hint at his impact on spine surgery.

Dr. Ray was co-founder of the North American Spine Society as well as the founding President of the Spine Arthroplasty Society (now known as the International Society for the Advancement of Spine Surgery), co-founder of the both the American College of Spine Surgery and the American Board of Spine Surgery.

Over his career Dr. Ray advised numerous firms including Hoffman-LaRoche in Basel, Switzerland, Medtronic, Inc. in Minneapolis, Minnesota and, of course, RayMedica Inc., in Minneapolis as well as InveRay, Ltd.

Charlie, as he was known by virtually everyone he came into contact with, held 53 U.S. patents and over 100 foreign patents, wrote over 365 articles and books and his bibliography lists 340 entries. He was the inventor of the Ray Threaded Fusion Cage, as well as the prosthetic nucleus to restore degenerative discs.

For this work he was declared the Gold Medal Winner of the Medical Design Excellence Award for the year 2000. He was also awarded one of the three R & D 100 (along with NASA and DuPont Inc.) Best of the Best Awards—his for the development of this product having the most humanistic application.

Charlie was born on August 1, 1927, in Americus, Georgia. a very small town about 130 miles southwest of Atlanta. In addition to Charlie Ray, Americus is the birthplace of Habitat for Humanity. Both Charlie and Habitat for Humanity would eventually become internationally known and renowned builders.

His parents, Oliver Tinsley Ray and Katherine Broadfield Ray, moved from Americus to Atlanta in 1937. There, Charlie attended the Technological High School and upon graduating in 1945 joined the U.S. Navy. With the Navy, Charlie began what would eventually become a lifetime of traveling the world. Over the course of the next 65 years, he trained surgeons on every continent, in hundreds of countries and became fluent in eight languages.

Charlie earned an undergraduate degree from Emory University in Atlanta and then a master's degree from the University of Miami in 1952. He earned his medical degree from the Medical College of Georgia in 1956 and completed his fellowship at the Mayo Clinic in Rochester, Minnesota. From there, Dr. Ray joined the staff at Johns Hopkins University taking the position of Assistant Professor of Neurosurgery and Bioengineering.

A Major Theoretical Influence

An expert in bioengineering, philosophy, medicine and biology, Dr. Ray was much more than just a surgeon engineer. He was a major theoretical influence on spine care because he championed arthrodesis and arthroplasty as treatment modalities for degenerative disc disease instead of fusion.

"Dr. Ray was one of the most creative men I ever met. He was not only a fantastically innovative and creative personality but most gracious and open to any and all queries. He would always be available to help with any and all ideas and always contributed more than his fair share. It was an honor to know Charlie and be able to call him a friend." — Stephen Hochschuler, M.D.

"Dr. Charles Ray, beside his impressive CV and his documented achievements, was a very warm and attentive man. Always innovating and inventing, ready to listen to problems and looking for solutions, he took on challenges that are daunting but needed to be initiated to benefit patients. He built consensus and led by example. He was an inventor, artist, writer and lecturer in five languages. Most importantly he was my friend." — Hansen A. Yuan, M.D.

"Charlie was a thought leader in the world of contemporary spine surgery. The Ray TFC cage changed how fusion surgery was performed. He was the first to address disc degeneration with a replacement for the degenerated nucleus. He was truly a pioneer as evidenced by so many arrows in his back. He invented to help patients." — John V. Viscogliosi, Viscogliosi Brothers, LLC

"Charlie Ray remains in my memory as a great human and a true pioneer of devices for the spine. My first contact with Charlie was in 2002 when I received a welcome letter from him on becoming a member of the Board of Directors of the Spine Arthroplasty Society. The Society had been formed a year earlier. Later I had the honor of cooperating with Charlie to revise the Society's bylaws and create today's ISASS, the International Society for the Advancement of Spine Surgery. I had many meetings and conversations with Charlie. He was an enjoyable gentleman and a good advisor. I will never forget him." — Karin Buettner-Janz, M.D., Ph.D.

Charles A. Rockwood Jr.

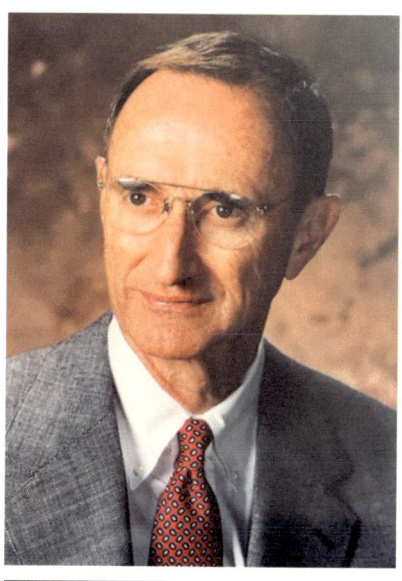

Born:	1929
Died:	2022
Years Active:	40+
Location:	San Antonia, TX
Role(s):	President of AAOS and OREF, Founder of the American Shoulder and Elbow Society, Chief of the Division of Orthopedics at University Texas Health Science Center and a pioneer orthopedic surgeon.

Charles A. Rockwood, Jr., M.D., former AAOS and OREF President, one of the founders of the American Shoulder and Elbow Society, is a pioneer in hip and knee surgery who influenced two generations of young orthopedic surgeons.

He was considered to be one of the premier shoulder surgeons in the world with young doctors from around the world vying for his fellowships. He was instrumental in the development of DePuy's Global Total Shoulder system which became the leading total shoulder arthroplasty system in the U.S. and the world. He implanted the first Global Shoulder system in the summer of 1990.

Rockwood was born in Oklahoma City on September 19, 1929, to Charles A. and Dorothy Rockwood. After graduating Classen High School in Oklahoma City and attending Oklahoma City University for pre-med studies, he did not initially get accepted into medical school.

He ended up spending a year on graduate studies before being accepted to the University of Oklahoma Medical School from which he graduated in 1956.

He then completed a one-year internship at Gorgas Hospital in the Panama Canal Zone before returning to Oklahoma City to serve in an Air Force-sponsored orthopedic surgery residency under the mentorship of Dr. Don O'Donoghue, pioneer knee surgeon and one of the fathers of American sports medicine.

After his residency, he spent five years at Wilford Hall Medical Center in San Antonio. He remained in the United States Air Force Reserve and retired as a Full Colonel.

In 1966, he became the third member of the surgical faculty at University Texas Health Science Center (now UT Health) in San Antonio. He then went on to serve as the Chief of the Division of Orthopaedics there.

Dr. Rockwood was also a past president of both the American Academy of Orthopaedic Surgeons and the Orthopaedic Research and Education Foundation. He was also an honorary fellow in the Royal College of Surgeons, Edinburgh, Scotland, and was recipient of the American-British Canadian Fellowship Award in 1967.

Christoph Röder

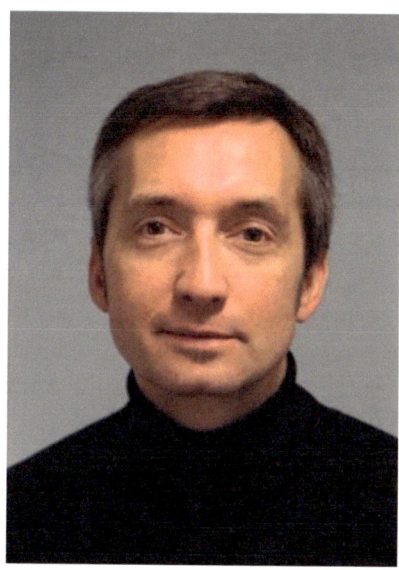

Born:	1971
Died:	2015
Years Active:	10+
Location:	Bern, Switzerland
Role(s):	Director of the Institute for Evaluative Research in Medicine and faculty member, University of Bern, Switzerland.

Christoph Röder, M.D., Ph.D., M.P.H., was director of the Institute for Evaluative Research in Medicine at the University of Bern in Switzerland and a senior researcher in Spine Tango, one of the first spine surgery registries in the world.

For 13 years, Christoph Röder led Spine Tango in an effort to ensure that reliable, comprehensive, and practice-changing data would be available to enhance spine care. Dr. Röder also spent time at the New York University Hospital for Joint Diseases, where he was a senior research fellow. Later, he was on the faculty at the University of Bern in Switzerland and then became the interim director and later the director of the Institute for Evaluative Research in Medicine at that facility.

Regarding Spine Tango, Dr. Röder was quoted as saying, "In the discussion about the rationale for spine registries, two basic questions have to be answered. The first one deals with the value of orthopaedic registries per se, considering them as observational studies and comparing the evidence they generate with that of randomized controlled trials. The second question asks if the need for registries in spine surgery is similar to that in the arthroplasty sector."

"The widely held view that randomized controlled trials are the 'gold standard' for evaluation and that observational methods have little, or no value ignores the limitations of randomised trials. They may prove unnecessary, inappropriate, impossible, or inadequate. In addition, the external validity and hence the ability to make generalisations about the results of randomised trials is often low."

"Therefore, the false conflict between those who advocate randomised trials in all situations and those who believe observational data provide sufficient evidence needs to be replaced with mutual recognition of their complementary roles."

"The fact that many surgical techniques or technologies were introduced into the field of spine surgery without randomised trials or prospective cohort comparisons makes obvious an even increased need for spine registries compared to joint arthroplasty. An essential methodological prerequisite for a registry is a common terminology for reporting results and a sophisticated technology that networks all participants so that one central data pool is created and accessed."

Zoher Ghogawala M.D., chairman of the Department of Neurosurgery at Tufts University School of Medicine said of Röder, "Chris Röder was a pioneer and champion of spinal registries. He passionately built the Spine Tango platform and shared his experience freely with others. He was ahead of his time and believed that global registries would ultimately improve spinal care. We are all benefitting from his leadership in the arena."

Emin Aghayev, M.D., a member of the Institute for Evaluative Research in Medicine at the University of Bern in Switzerland said of Dr. Röder, "He made outcome research and development of medical registries his aim in life. One of his major projects was the international Spine Tango registry that has grown to over 85,000 surgery forms and 220, 000 patient-based COMI forms from over 50 spine centers in 17 European and Non-European countries, and that has published about 45 peer-reviewed articles."

Leon Root

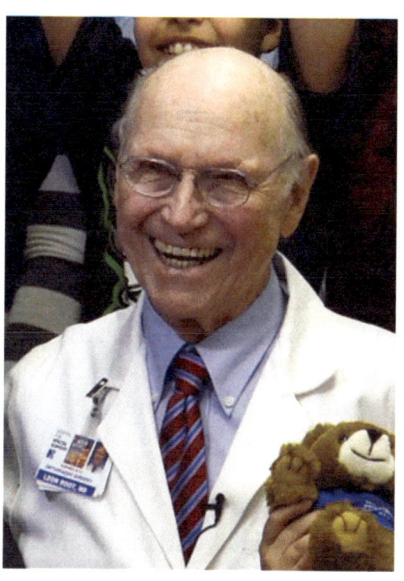

Born:	1928
Died:	2015
Years Active:	50+
Location:	New York City
Role(s):	Chief of Pediatric Orthopedics at the Hospital for Special Surgery, Founded NYC's first osteogenesis imperfecta clinic, founded first Pediatric Orthopedic Outreach program in New York, President of the American Academy for Cerebral Palsy and Developmental Medicine

Leon Root, M.D., pioneered many pediatric orthopedic initiatives notably New York City's first osteogenesis imperfecta clinic, the first Pediatric Orthopedic Outreach program in New York and then served as President of the American Academy for Cerebral Palsy and Developmental Medicine, For 47 years, when nervous children and families awaited their appointments at Hospital for Special Surgery (HSS), their fears were eased when Leon Root reached out to greet them. Dr. Root was the talented and pioneering chief of pediatric orthopedics at New York City's Hospital for Special Surgery for 27 years.

Only three years after joining HSS in 1968, Dr. Root established New York City's first clinic for children with osteogenesis imperfecta (OI), a congenital bone disorder characterized by brittle bones that are prone to fracture. People with OI are born with defective connective tissue, or without the ability to produce the tissue, usually because of a deficiency of type I collagen.

When Dr. Root recognized how difficult it was for many of the city's children to come to him, he went to them, establishing the state's first Pediatric Orthopedic Outreach Program (POP). Because of Dr. Root's efforts, more than 26, 000 children have been screened in New York schools; 4, 000 of those children were referred for further medical care.

Lou Shapiro, CEO of HSS, said this of Dr. Root, "My memorable moment of Dr. Root was actually captured in a beautiful photo of Dr. Root surrounded by smiling children from a school in the Bronx in New York. Dr. Root and a team of residents, fellows, nurses and members of our Education staff had just conducted the HSS POP school screening. The moment and photo speak volumes about Dr. Root. He was truly an outstanding person and physician that embodied the overall mission of HSS—to serve and care for the community. It is who he was and how he lived."

Dr. Root expanded the HSS Cerebral Palsy Clinic and served as president of the American Academy for Cerebral Palsy and Developmental Medicine.

On the research front, Dr. Root helped found what is now known as the Leon Root Motion Analysis Laboratory.

When Dr. Root first joined the Hospital for Special Surgery, there were only eight orthopedic surgeons at that institution. Joint arthroplasty and other advanced diagnosis and treatment modalities were just emerging. Over his career at HSS, the surgical staff grew by 12-fold to more than 100 board certified surgeons.

Dr. Root was one of the United States foremost specialists in pediatric orthopedics

Dr. Cathleen Raggio, a pediatric orthopedic surgeon at HSS, said this about Dr. Root, "Dr. Root is the reason I went into orthopedic surgery 30 years ago. I met him when I was a third-year medical student."

"When I told him I had already decided to do a pediatrics internship but now wanted to go into orthopedics and would have to do two internships, I said I hope that that's not going to be a problem. He said, 'That's not a problem—this is great news! You're going to do well. So what, you have to do two internships. It'll be fine.' That's typical of Dr. Root—he turned everything into a positive and really encouraged you to do your best."

"Dr. Root was very inquisitive. He would ask questions and always listened to the answers. That's a very important quality. He not only asked "why" but he listened to what other people might suggest. Then he would follow through, think about it and research it."

Leon Root attended Rutgers University, earning a Bachelor of Science degree in 1951. He obtained his medical degree from New York Medical College in 1955 and interned as a general practitioner at Beth Israel Hospital in Newark, New Jersey. He completed his residency at St. Joseph's Hospital in Paterson, New Jersey, and then accepted a one-year fellowship at the Hospital for Special Surgery, where he remained for the rest of his career.

Richard Rothman

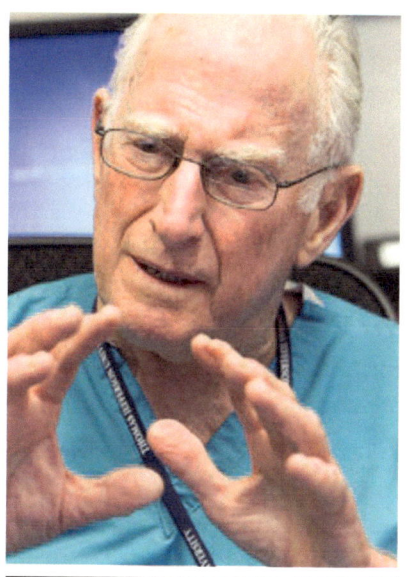

Richard Rothman, M.D., Ph.D., is the founder of the Rothman Institute in Philadelphia, which has clinics in Pennsylvania, New Jersey, and New York, provides team physicians for the Philadelphia-based professional sports teams—Phillies, Eagles, Flyers, and 76ers—as well as those of national NCAA basketball champions Villanova University.

The Rothman Institute is one of the largest and most influential orthopedic and spine care networks in the world with more than 200 physicians in over 30 offices and managing three quarters of a million patient visits annually.

During his long and remarkable career, Dr. Rothman has personally performed over 50,000 total hip and knee arthroplasty procedures. Dr. Rothman also developed the Stryker Accolade total hip replacement system, which has become one of the most prominent and widely used hip replacement systems in the world.

Born in nearby Cheltenham, Pennsylvania, he majored in history at the University of Pennsylvania, then obtained a Ph.D. in anatomy from Thomas Jefferson University in Philadelphia.

After earning an M.D. from the Perelman School of Medicine at the University of Pennsylvania in 1962, Dr. Rothman returned to Jefferson for a residency.

Seven years out of medical school, Richard Rothman boarded a plane to England and made the trek to Sir John Charnley's lab and learned the, then new hip arthroplasty procedure.

Born:	1937
Died:	2018
Years Active:	53
Location:	Philadelphia, PA
Role(s):	Joint arthroplasty pioneer, trained with Sir John Charnley, founder of the Rothman Institute, Professor of Orthopedic Surgery, Vice Chairman of the Board of Trustees at Thomas Jefferson University

So impressed was Dr. Charnley with Richard Rothman's talent that when Walter Annenberg, the publisher of Reader's Digest and also a Philadelphia resident, sought out Charnley for hip surgery, Charley pointed him back to his own neighborhood...and to Dr. Rothman.

Annenberg, pleased with the results of two hip surgeries performed by Dr. Rothman, donated millions of dollars that set the stage for the Rothman Institute.

Michael G. Ciccotti, M.D., director of the Sports Medicine Team at the Rothman Orthopaedic Institute said of Dr. Rothman, "Dr. Rothman started out as chairman of Thomas Jefferson University orthopedics in 1986, my first year of practice. I was his intern, I did my residency with him, and then joined the practice. He was a beacon of wisdom and goodwill for my entire orthopedic career."

"Not only was he a wonderful, true friend, Dick had the gift of making the most complex issues—whether practice management, medical, or interpersonal—very understandable. He instinctively knew how to remove the emotion from any situation and guide us toward the best solution."

Alex Vaccaro, President of the Rothman Institute, said, "Many people don't know this about Dick, but he was a consummate businessman. Although he retired from the operating room in May 2018, he continued to pursue his passion for helping companies succeed, even working with Wall Street because he was so knowledgeable about the world of orthopedics. He was a senior advisor to The Riverside Company and HealthpointCapital."

Richard Rothman was the founder and acting Chairman of the Board of Specialty Care Network, a publicly held company now known as Healthgrades. He served on multiple corporate boards and was an advisor for the Washington, D.C.-based Carlyle Group.

Dr. Rothman also looked beyond the borders of the U.S., devoting many hours to teaching assignments in China, India and Korea.

Dr. Vaccaro notes, "Dick was determined to establish the Rothman level of quality abroad and was spearheading our efforts to collaborate with health systems in China, Italy, and Dubai."

Dr. Rothman served as the Editor-in-Chief and then Emeritus Editor of *The Journal of Arthroplasty*, the most widely read peer-reviewed journal dedicated to total joint replacement. He published more than 200 original research papers and over 15 orthopedic textbooks on spine and joint replacement surgery.

His dedication to advancing the quality of what was available to patients led to the development of the Accolade total hip system (now made by Stryker Corporation), which has been used in over 200,000 patients to date.

Dr. Rothman was also active in the development improvement of highly cross-linked polyethylene bearings including Crossfire and X3, as well as the continued development of the Trident shell.

He served as Vice Chairman of the Board of Trustees at Thomas Jefferson University. Previously, he was on the Board of the American Academy of Orthopaedic Surgeons and was a trustee at the College of General Studies, University of Pennsylvania and the Brandywine Museum.

He received the Sir John Charnley Award for outstanding service and achievement in total joint replacement, as well as the Frank Stinchfield Award from the Hip Society.

A fan of the Rolling Stones, Rothman often said, "You can't always get what you want...but if you try sometimes, well you just might find, you get what you need."

Mitchell Seyedin

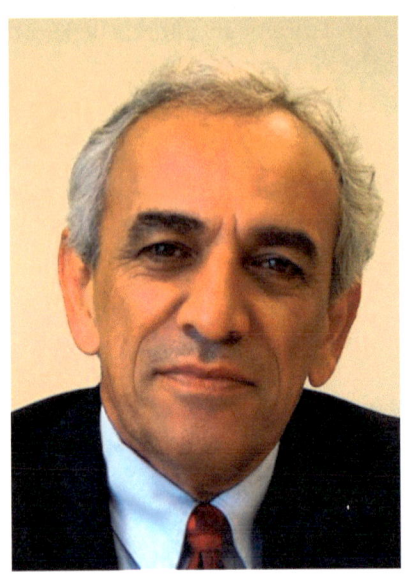

Born:	1948
Died:	2014
Years Active:	40+
Location:	St. Louis, MO
Role(s):	Pioneer and global leader in the field of regenerative medicine. Founder of such seminal regenerative medicine companies as Orquest, Metra Biosystems and ISTO Technologies.

Mitchell Seyedin, Ph.D., one of the pioneers in regenerative medicine for orthopedics and, most recently, Chief Scientific Officer and Executive Chairman of ISTO Technologies, Inc.

His infectious enthusiasm for the science of regenerative medicine inspired thousands of physicians and orthopedic executives to join him in the great march to regenerative healing and in many ways fueled the development of this entire industry.

Dr. Seyedin received an undergraduate degree in chemistry from the University of Wisconsin, River Falls, and a Ph.D. in biological chemistry from the University of South Carolina, Columbia. He was also a Postdoctoral Research Fellow at the University of California, Berkeley.

Mitch Seyedin was an innovator in the truest sense of that word. Prior to leading ISTO, he was co-founder, president, and chief executive officer of CBYON, a medical technology company that developed and marketed advanced visualization and navigation systems for minimally invasive surgery.

Before CBYON he founded Orquest, Inc., a bone and cartilage tissue engineering company that is now a key part of the DePuy unit of Johnson & Johnson. Dr. Seyedin was president and chief executive officer until 1996, and chairman and chief scientific officer until 1999. Earlier in his career, Dr. Seyedin co-founded Metra Biosystems, Inc., a diagnostic company that went public in 1995 and was acquired by Quidel in 1999.

Mitch rose to national prominence early in his career when he served as director of the Cellular Biochemistry Department at Collagen Corporation, where he was responsible for all aspects of tissue engineering and growth factor research programs and was awarded 11 patents.

Scott Gill of ISTO Technologies said of Dr. Seyedin, "He balanced his exceptionally strong scientific mind with a keen sense for business but also a true compassion for the well-being of those that worked for and with him. Anyone that had the pleasure of knowing him or working with him is better off for that experience."

Joseph Lane, M.D. of Hospital for Special Surgery said, "I remember Mitch when he was a recent Ph.D. graduate. He was working at Collagen Corporation and pretty much single handedly developed Collagraft. He was an extraordinary investigator and his skills and determination have been evident throughout his illustrious career. It is an honor and a pleasure to have been friends with Mitch."

Russell E. Windsor

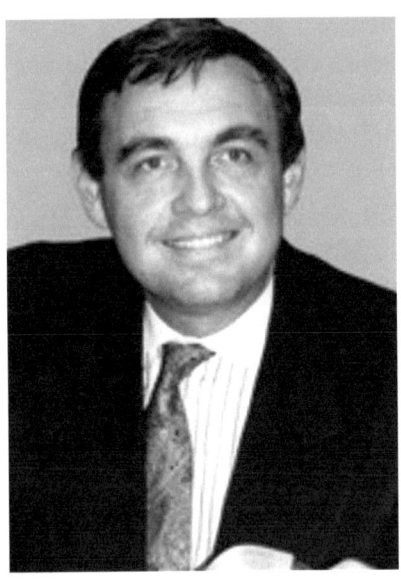

Born:	1952
Died:	2022
Years Active:	
Location:	New York City
Role(s):	Knee replacement pioneer, Professor of Orthopedic Surgery Weill Cornell Medicine, President of the Knee Society, designer of innovative and widely used knee implants

Russell E. Windsor, M.D., was a pioneer in knee replacement surgery, Professor of orthopedic surgery, President of the Knee Society designer of innovative and widely used knee implants and instrument.

Windsor was fascinated with medicine at a young age and could be found studying anatomy textbooks for fun as a child. He was very passionate about helping others and always knew he wanted to be a physician.

An integral moment in his medical education was when he did a fellowship under John Insall, M.D. chief of the Hospital for Special Surgery in New York, founding member of The Knee Society and one of the original fathers of total knee replacement surgery.

Windsor went on to have his own significant impact on the field of orthopedic surgery. He was a designer of several innovative and widely used total knee replacement systems, including the Rotating Hinge Knee and the Zimmer Unicompartmental Knee. Throughout his medical career, he was especially interested in surgical applications of computer-assisted navigation and robotics in knee replacement and the treatment of complex deformities of the knee.

For over 35 years, he was an attending orthopedic surgeon in the Adult Reconstruction & Joint Replacement Surgery Service at Hospital for Special Surgery in New York City. He also served as a professor of orthopedic surgery at Weill Cornell Medicine for more than 25 years and was chief of the knee service from 1991 to 2006.

Windsor was a member of the International Society of Arthroscopy Knee Surgery and Orthopaedic Sports Medicine, the American Association of Hip and Knee Surgeons, the American Academy of Orthopaedic Surgeons, and the American Knee Society. He served as president of the American Knee Society in 2005. He was also an international member of the European Knee Society.

Educating younger generations of orthopedic surgeons was important to Windsor. He wrote over 60 original publications and contributed chapters in 40 textbooks. He also presented his work and served as faculty member in over 250 national and international seminars.

Windsor spent 15 years helping to train orthopedic and trauma surgeons in Eastern Europe through the American Austrian Foundation Salzburg Seminars, Open Medical Institute. He also mentored hundreds of residents and fellows before retiring in 2021.

Windsor was born on March 13, 1952, to Alberta and Russell W. Windsor in Philadelphia, Pennsylvania. He attended LaSalle High School, and then Georgetown University for his bachelor's degree and his medical degree. He went on to the University of Pennsylvania for his orthopaedic surgery residency and Hospital for Special Surgery for a fellowship in knee reconstructive surgery.

Music was also a passion of Windsor's. He was an accomplished classical pianist and loved listening to orchestral classical music. His favorite composers were Bruckner, Rachmaninoff, and Beethoven. He supported both Carnegie Hall and the Salzburg Music Festival.

Always active, he loved playing, and coaching and watching his favorite sports, baseball, rowing, and cycling. A wine connoisseur, he had a collection of over 4,000 bottles from all over the world and was a member of the New York chapter of the Confrerie des Chevaliers du Tastevin.

Willem Zeegers

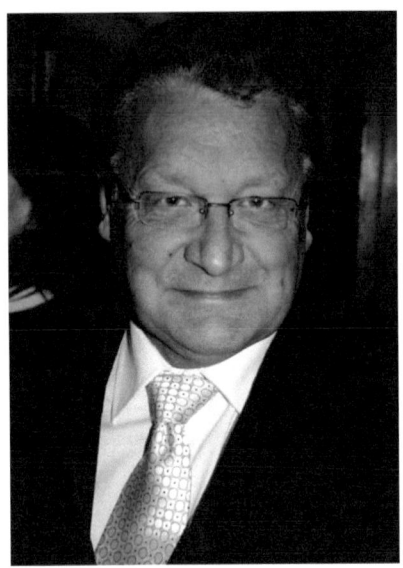

Born:	1945
Died:	2017
Years Active:	
Location:	Maastricht, Limburg, Netherlands
Role(s):	Artificial disc replacement pioneer

Dr. Willem Zeegers was a controversial pioneer of total disc replacement (TDR)/artificial disc replacement (ADR.

He performed one of the very first total disc replacements in 1989. Spine disc arthroplasty, like many other orthopedic and spine innovations came from a group of brilliant, talented and, occasionally, aggressive European surgeons and engineers, like Dr. Zeegers.

As part of that formative group, Dr. Zeegers became one of the leading lecturers and instructors in this novel procedure for more than 20 years.

Born on April 11, 1945, in Maastricht, Netherlands, Willem Zeegers came to devote his life to medicine, becoming an orthopaedic surgeon and inventor. He was one of the first surgeons to use STALIF (standalone lumbar fusion) and then, later to use, design, teach and consult about the spine disc arthroplasty and the use of Artificial Disc Replacements.

Dr. Zeeger earned his medical degree in Amsterdam in 1973. From 1973 – 1976 he practiced General Surgery at Onze Lieve Vrouwe Gasthuis in Amsterdam. He completed an Orthopaedic residency at St.Lucas & Binnengasthuis, also in Amsterdam. In 1980, he became registered as orthopaedic surgeon.

From 1980 – 1983 Dr. Zeeger's was the general Orthopaedic Consultant for Atrium Hospital in Heerlen, and then from 1983 – 2000, he was at Maasland Hospital in Sittard.

From 2000 – 2008 he was a Consultant Spinal Surgery at the Alpha Klinik in Munich.

In 2008 he became a global consultant in artificial disc replacement.

A longtime friend, Roberto Posavec, said, of Dr. Zeeger, "His special contribution is definitely in [the] field of TDR/ADR...many surgeons from the U.S. started ADR surgery after watching Willem (for example Texas Back Institute). Willem started with ADR in 1989."

"About 25 years ago Willem visited Zagreb, Croatia. He was invited to perform first the lumbar artificial disc replacement (ADR) in Croatia. The event organizer invited politicians, the mayor, and several journalists to cover this story. When Willem arrived, he found that he had been tricked. It was not the patient he was supposed to operate on. *This* patient did not have clear indications for ADR, so Willem turned around and left the hospital!"

"Willem was a consummate instructor, and unselfishly shared his knowledge and wisdom with physicians from around the globe. In his career he performed over 3,100 implantations of artificial discs."

One of the first patients to ever receive a total disc arthroplasty said this about Dr. Zeegers, "The first time I came for a treatment was in 1986 and Dr. Zeegers noticed immediately that my back was in bad condition after an operation by another surgeon."

"Dr. Zeeger worked for three years on a solution for my back, before he decided in 1989 to implant two artificial discs. I was the first patient for this kind of operation. I will never forget that Dr. Zeeger sat on my bed, talking to me, explaining the whole operation after he had to cancel it two times."

"He was so confident that it would be possible, that is was the best solution. That is why I can still walk, even he performed five surgeries after this operation, but it was necessary. Dr. Zeeger was a great lovely person who really cared about his patients."

From 1989, when he performed his first total disc replacement, to 2009, Dr. Zeegers taught, developed and wrote about Artificial Disc Replacement (ADR) surgery. He used ADR for as many as three spine levels. Because of his experience as a surgeon and taking advantage of the evolutionary improvements of implants, overall success rates under his hands, he reported, were > 87%.

Regional Founders, Pioneers *and* Champions of Modern Orthopedic *and* Spine Surgery

Albert Bernard Accettola

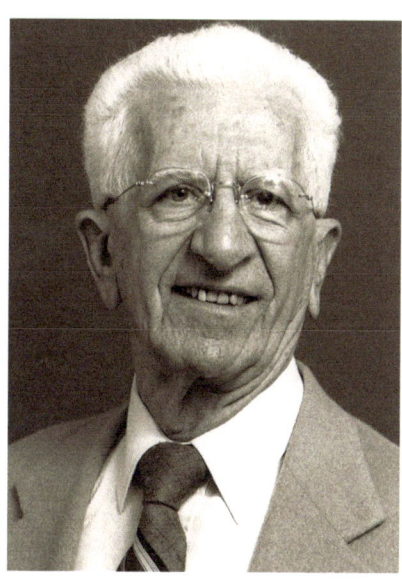

Born:	1918
Died:	2017
Years Active:	43
Location:	Staten Island, NY
Role(s):	Founder of Ortho Department Marquette University and Hunterdon Medical Center

Dr. Accettola was one of the founders of Marquette University and Hunterdon Medical Center's Department of Orthopedics. He also held positions at Staten Island University Hospital and Bellevue Hospital.

Dr. Accettola taught orthopedics as an associate clinical professor at New York University and was the orthopedic surgeon to all athletic teams at Wagner College from 1949 to 1987.

Dr. Accettola was a member and past president of the Richmond County Medical Society, a past president of the Medical Board of Staten Island University Hospital, and an active member of the New York State Medical Society, serving on numerous committees.

Albert Accettola was born on February 4, 1918, in New York City. He graduated from Wagner College in 1940 and then attended Boston University Medical School, where he graduated in 1944.

A fencer during his undergraduate years, Wagner College wrote of Dr. Accettola: "Whether with a saber in his hand or a scalpel, Al Accettola has been a gift to Wagner sports."

Noel Testa, M.D., clinical professor of orthopaedic surgery at NYU Langone Health, stated, "I knew Dr. Accettola as an attending in the Department of Orthopaedics during my residency. He was a gentleman in the truest sense of the word."

"Dr. Accettola was a dedicated educator, a talented diagnostician and a skilled orthopaedic surgeon. He was well liked and respected by his peers and his students."

"He brought quality orthopaedic care to the borough of Staten Island when it was only connected to the rest of New York City by the Staten Island Ferry."

Dan Adair

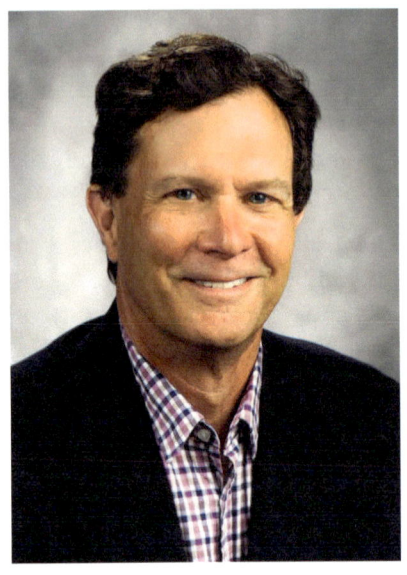

Born:	1954
Died:	2015
Years Active:	30+
Location:	Springfield, IL
Role(s):	Medical Director of Orthopedic Services, Memorial Medical Center. Co-Director of Orthopedics at Springfield Clinic and SportsCare of Illinois.

Dan Adair, M.D., was Medical Director of Orthopedic Services at Memorial Medical Center, Co-Director of the Orthopedic Group at Springfield Clinic, and Co-Medical Director at SportsCare of Illinois.

Dr. Adair was a strong advocate, both regionally and nationally, for a statistic driven approach towards adopting uniform methodologies for removing inefficiencies and improving overall procedure success rates. His advocacy in this area has continued through the work of many others.

Dr. Adair earned his medical degree at Southern Illinois University School of Medicine in Springfield, Illinois.

Through his 30 years of orthopedic service, Dr. Adair built an outstanding orthopedic group, three sports medicine programs, and fostered a new era in orthopedics at the Springfield Clinic and Memorial.

He trained over 90 residents and countless medical and nursing students. Through his leadership he took his Central Illinois Orthopedic Group from 3 orthopedic surgeons to 15, 3 podiatrists and 3 primary care sports medicine providers, 10 mid-levels, and 3 surgical assists.

At the time of his passing, he was the Co-Chairman of the Orthopedic Group at Springfield Clinic, while serving on numerous AAOS committees.

"Over his last few years, Dr. Adair also dedicated a significant amount of his energies towards improving the quality of care offered to orthopedic patients everywhere.

Dr. Adair began his professional career as an intern and resident at the Bowman-Gray School of Medicine at Wake Forest University."

Dr. Brett Wolters, an orthopedic surgeon at Springfield Clinic, described Dr. Dan Adair, "I always thought of him as a doctor, but I also thought of him as a leader, a visionary, a mentor and a dear friend."

I was fortunate to have met him in medical school. He was the one that convinced me to do orthopedics, he was the one that convinced me to do sports medicine. I thrived on doing cases with him, even if it was a simple total knee. It was his ability and ease at teaching me as well as making me feel capable. He was never in a rush. It was because of my experiences with Dan that I joined the Springfield Clinic.

Pete Stoll, Sports Medicine Coordinator at Springfield Clinic Sports Medicine, remembers, "It was the 1985 football season, and I was Dan's athletic trainer, providing field coverage at local Friday night prep games."

"Dan came into the office one Monday morning and said he'd gotten a concerned call from one of his partners in the Family Practice Department who wanted to know who that was on the field Friday night. The family doctor told Dan that Sports Medicine was just a 'gimmick' to divert patients from his office to the orthopedist's. Dan simply told him, 'If you tell me you'll be at every high school football game, I'll pull my trainer off the field.' That was the end of the discussion.

Thirty years later, Springfield has several local sports medicine programs, which Dan Adair helped create, and numerous athletic trainers covering nearly every varsity practice and game at high schools and colleges throughout the region. There's no question in my mind that Dan Adair was the Father of Sports Medicine in the area. He transformed a 'gimmick' to one of the most successful and respected medical programs in central Illinois."

"Dan would probably like to be remembered as a great surgeon, mentor and friend. He was intently focused on measuring performance and continually improving outcomes. He used his skills where they were most needed—first in the Sports Medicine arena, then later to help keep an aging boomer population active.

Dan didn't stop at the clinical aspects of his role as an orthopedic surgeon. He was a tremendous mentor to so many area orthopedic surgeons. He was a tremendous athlete in his own right—not just talking the talk, but walking the walk as a tennis player, cyclist, runner and triathlete. Dan was a loving husband, and proud father and grandfather. He was a great friend and colleague."

Frank J. Boutin Sr.

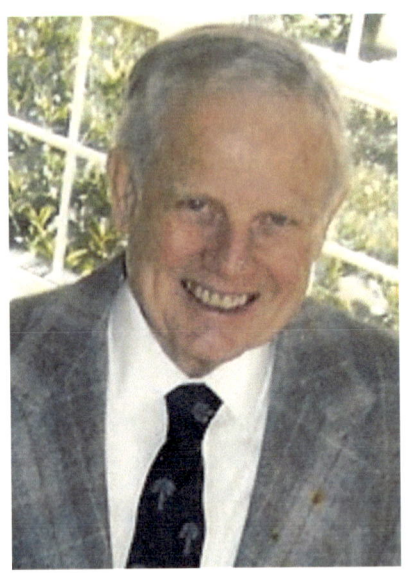

Born:	1920
Died:	2013
Years Active:	40+
Location:	Sacramento, CA
Role(s):	"Father of Orthopedics" in Sacramento, California

Frank J. Boutin Sr. was one of the first orthopedic surgeons in Sacramento. "He dispensed a lot of good advice about setting up practices; in fact, he was the 'go-to' guy in this respect. He was the quintessential gentleman surgeon," said Robert Szabo, M.D. a longtime colleague.

Born on June 9, 1920, in Spokane, Washington, Dr. Boutin went on to earn his undergraduate degree from Stanford University in 1942. He then enlisted in the Army, attended Stanford Medical School, and then served at Walter Reed Army Medical Center in Washington, D.C.

After his Army service, Dr. Boutin and his family headed back to the West Coast where he served as chief resident at Stanford University Hospital and San Francisco General Hospital. In 1953, the family moved to Woodland, California, so that Dr. Boutin could become the first orthopedic surgeon at the Woodland Clinic.

According to David Coward, M.D., one of Dr. Boutin's colleagues, "He devoted over 40 years to caring for patients and mentoring all new orthopedic surgeons. He had a tremendous influence on the entire orthopedic community in Sacramento. He set the bar at a high level for all of us. Dr. Frank J. Boutin, Sr. was a great man, a wonderful friend, and an amazing orthopedic surgeon."

"Frank would never drink alcohol 72 hours before any planned surgical procedure. And to take it one step further, he would not drink for 72 hours if there was even a chance, he might be performing surgery."

"Dr. Boutin began his medical career caring for World War II soldiers with orthopedic wounds and training under Sterling Bunnell, the Father of Hand Surgery. But his career also included a wide array of other orthopedic subspecialties, including pediatric orthopedics, spine, arthroplasty, and arthroscopy. Constantly training to learn new techniques/information as it came along was extremely important to him."

According to those who knew him best, one aspect of Dr. Boutin, a child of the Great Depression, that stood above all others was his sense of duty.

David Lance Bowles

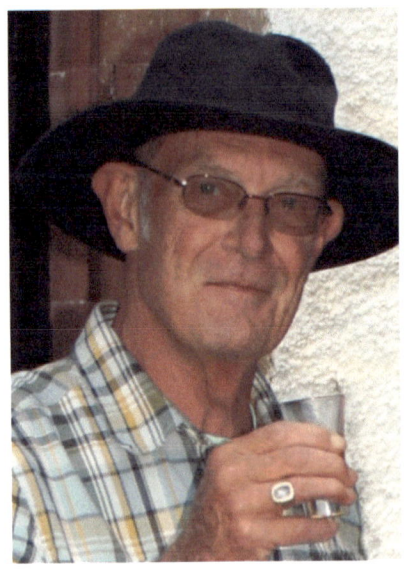

David Lance Bowles, M.D., of Streetman, Texas was a pioneering orthopedic surgeon when, in June 1982, he broke new ground as the only orthopedic surgeon in east Texas, Henderson County, population of just 10,000 people. His solo practice was in Athens, Texas.

Bowles was born in Tulsa, Oklahoma, on June 29, 1951, to Norma and William R. Bowles. He grew up in Bartlesville, Oklahoma, where he graduated from Sooner High School in 1969. He went on to earn his bachelor's degree from Oklahoma State University. He completed his medical degree in 1977 from the University of Texas Southwestern Medical School.

After completing a general surgery internship at Methodist Hospital of Dallas, he then did a four-year orthopedic surgery residency at John Peter Smith Hospital in Fort Worth, Texas. He served East Texas patients for more than 36 years.

Born:	1951
Died:	2022
Years Active:	36
Location:	East Texas
Role(s):	Pioneer orthopedic surgeon

Glenn Blish Carpenter

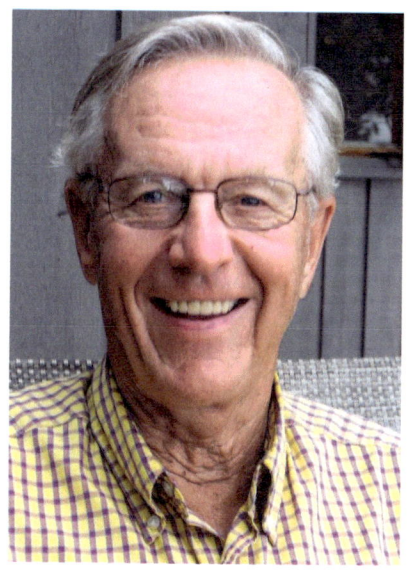

Born:	1926
Died:	2022
Years Active:	40+
Location:	Detroit, MI
Role(s):	Pioneer orthopedic surgeon. President of the Oakland County Medical Society.

Dr. Glenn Blish Carpenter, one of the first arthroplasty surgeons in Detroit, Michigan. He also served in the Pacific Theater during World War II and spent more than 40 years in the Beaumont Hospital system.

Dr. Carpenter earned his medical degree from the University of Michigan Medical School in 1953 and began his orthopedic training at the University of Michigan. He entered orthopedic practice just before joint arthroplasty surgery became a standard of care for osteoarthritic or fractured joints.

Dr. Carpenter began his practice in Birmingham, Michigan, on the staff at Beaumont Hospital in Royal Oak, Michigan where he would stay for more than 40 years. Eventually, Dr. Carpenter's sterling reputation as a physician led to his election as president of the Oakland County Medical Society.

He served his country during World War II and then came home to finish his undergraduate studies and follow his father into medicine.

He especially enjoyed the Detroit Institute of Arts, the Detroit Symphony, and Cranbrook Schools. Both the arts and sciences were important to him.

Dr. Carpenter was born in 1926 in Detroit, Michigan to Glenn B. and Grace Carpenter. He grew up on the famous Seven Mile Road and attended Hampton and Cranbrook Schools.

Robert C. Coddington

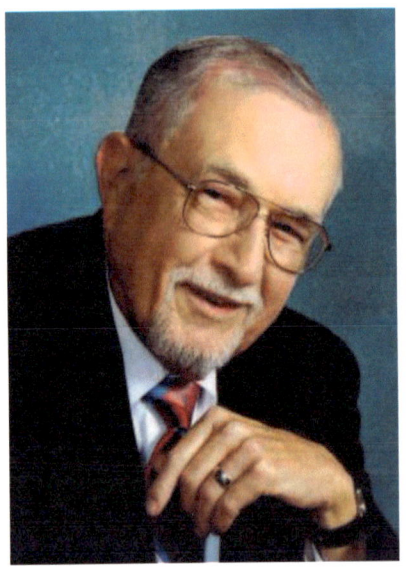

Born:	1932
Died:	2021
Years Active:	42
Location:	Chattanooga-Hixon, TN
Role(s):	Chair, University of Tennessee College of Medicine at Chattanooga, Past president Tennessee Orthopaedic Society

Robert C. Coddington, M.D., was chair of the University of Tennessee College of Medicine at Chattanooga from 1974 to 1996. He also served as that institution's associate dean and professor from 1974 to 1983. Dr. Coddington was instrumental in bringing the medical school to Chattanooga.

For 15 years Dr. Coddington was the board examiner for the American Orthopedic Society and he was a fellow with the American Academy of Orthopaedic Surgeons and the American College of Surgeons.

Dr. Coddington was also the former president of the Tennessee Orthopaedic Society and a founding member of the Southeast Tennessee Area Health Education Center.

In total, Dr. Coddington served the Chattanooga-Hixon, Tennessee, communities for more than four decades, 1967 to 2009 when he retired.

His started in private practice with the Chattanooga Orthopaedic Group and then went solo in 1974 specializing in pediatric and adolescent orthopedic surgery.

Dr. Coddington was known for his dedication to developing and supporting orthopedic residents as well as physician assistants.

He was very involved in the community. He held the Crippled Children's Clinic at T.C. Thompson Children's Hospital for 25 years and donated his expertise to children in need through the state's Crippled Children's Clinic. He held the position of team physician for various Kirkman and Hixon high schools as well.

Born on August 30, 1931, he spent his early years in LaPorte, Indiana. He received his medical degree from the Indiana University Medical Center, where he went on to complete his orthopedic residency training program.

Dr. Coddington served in the U.S. Army from 1962 to 1966 and later served in the Tennessee Army National Guard. He received the Army Commendation Medal, Meritorious Service Medal and the Legion of Merit. He retired with the rank of Colonel.

Frank F. Cook

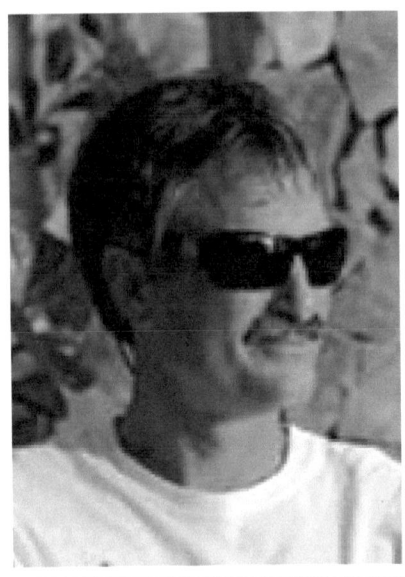

Frank Cook was the co-founder of Palm Beach Orthopedics Institute and served as its president for 10 years. Dr. Cook was also orthopedic consultant to the four major league baseball teams – the Florida Marlins, Montreal Expos, St. Louis Cardinals, and Los Angeles Dodgers.

For nearly 25 years, Dr. Cook was an orthopedic surgeon at Jupiter Medical Center (JMC).

Frank Cook completed his orthopedic surgery residency at University Hospital (Shands) in Jacksonville, Florida. In the mid-1980s, he completed a sports medicine fellowship at the Kerlan-Jobe Clinic.

Richard K. Ryu M.D., Surgical Director for Summit and Premier Surgery Centers in Santa Barbera, California said, "As co-fellows at the Kerlan-Jobe Orthopaedic Clinic, Dr. Cook was not only a gifted surgeon, but as one of the genuinely funniest and most irreverent people I have had the pleasure of knowing. His sartorial splendor is best described as 'Miami Vice visits Los Angeles'. Always armed with a kind word for those he worked with, and quick with a quip or smile, collaborating and training with Frank was nothing short of delightful."

Born:	1955
Died:	2014
Years Active:	30+
Location:	Jupiter, FL
Role(s):	Co-Founder Palm Beach Orthopedics Institute and President of the Institute for 10 years.

James E. Tibone, M.D. professor of clinical orthopaedic surgery at the Keck School of Medicine of USC, and the 2018 Robert E. Leach Sports Medicine Leadership Award winner, said, "Frank was one of our best sports fellows. Very smart. Great surgeon and clinician with good hands."

Frank Cook attended the University of Florida where he majored in Biochemistry and continued into medical school at the same institution, receiving his M.D in 1980. His devotion to medicine was inspired by a singular incident at Blue Springs,

Florida, when, as an undergraduate, he rescued and resuscitated a diver. Frank knew then that he would devote his life to helping others through medicine."

"His passion for physical fitness training as well as multiple sports—running, biking, swimming, baseball—made Frank ideally suited for orthopedic medicine. An athlete himself, Frank understood his patients' frustration with the recovery process and their impatience to return to the arena. Dressed in one of his trademark Hawaiian shirts for office visits, he was at one with the passion that drove his patients to push themselves."

John D. Couris, president, and chief executive officer of Jupiter Medical Center, said, "Dr. Cook was an immensely talented surgeon who was deeply respected by his patients and his peers. His dedication and leadership helped transform Jupiter Medical Center into the world-class facility that it is today.

Eugene "Gene" R. Corasanti

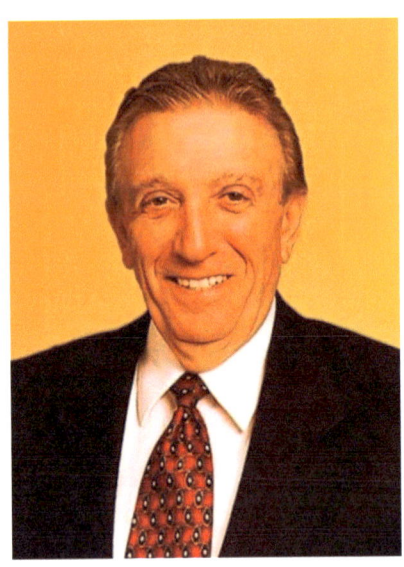

Born:	1931
Died:	2015
Years Active:	36
Location:	Utica, NY
Role(s):	Founder and CEO of the CONMED corporation, medical manufacturing visionary and industry leader.

Eugene R. Corasanti, known as the gentlemanly founder of CONMED Corporation – one of the pioneering suppliers of minimally invasive instruments and equipment.

Corasanti, who'd graduated Magna Cum Laude in accounting from Niagara University, founded the Consolidated Medical Equipment company in 1970 – changing the name later to CONMED.

Corasanti served as CEO and Chairman of the Board from 1970 to his retirement in 2006. CONMED, which sold approximately $1 billion of surgical and patient monitoring products in 2022 and is valued at nearly $2.5 billion, is one of the most admired companies in medicine. And a major reason for that is Gene Corasanti – or as he was also known: "The Gentleman CEO".

Robert Shallish, Jr., CONMED's former Chief Financial Officer said, "Gene was a strong believer in detailed risk/reward analysis. When analyzing a particular course of action, he would always say, 'Don't tell me how much I can make, tell me how much I could lose.' This credo allowed the company to be rewarded through acceptance of reasonable risk without taking extreme bets."

"Through Gene's persistence, he created an organization from scratch focused on providing important medical devices to the healthcare community, while at the same time creating value for shareholders and meaningful opportunity to thousands of employees. He accomplished this while being a true gentleman who recognized the personal self-worth of every individual he met."

Shortly after graduating from Niagara University, Corasanti served in the U.S.

Army and was stationed at the U.S. Finance Center in St. Louis, Missouri. Corasanti began his career as an independent public accountant, working at Brooks, Sugarman & Cone for many years.

"Gene was a true 'Gentleman' in every sense of the word and admired by many," wrote the Utica Observer Dispatch newspaper.

David C. Cottrell II

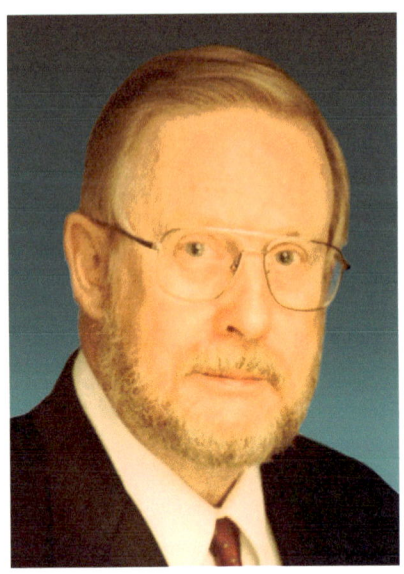

Born:	1933
Died:	2020
Years Active:	38+
Location:	Philadelphia, PA
Role(s):	Professor of orthopedic surgery, University of Pennsylvania

David C. Cottrell, II, M.D was a professor of orthopedic surgery at the University of Pennsylvania and longtime orthopedic surgeon in the Philadelphia region.

Dr. Cottrell entered orthopedics and, later, the faculty at one of the premier medical schools in the world, at the time when large joint and extremity arthroplasty was entering the standard of care in modern medicine.

Although a native of Philadelphia. Cottrell chose the University of Tennesee for his undergraduate work – earning BA in 1955. He did return to Philadelphia from Knoxville and earned his medical degree from University of Pennsylvania School of Medicine in 1959. Cottrell subsequently completed both his internship and residency at the Hospital of the University of Pennsylvania.

With his medical degree, Cottrell served as a captain in the Army and for a time was stationed in Okinawa, Japan. He was honorably discharged in 1962.

Also in 1962, Dr. Cottrell was invited to join the faculty at the University of Pennsylvania as an assistant instructor and research fellow in orthopedic surgery. The next year he was appointed assistant instructor and resident and, later, to be appointed associate clinical educator, finally clinical assistant professor in 1980.

Dr. Cottrell maintained a private in Bryn Mawr Hospital. In 1986, he opened another practice in Selinsgrove, Pennsylvania, performing surgery at the Evangelical Community Hospital in Lewisburg and at the Sunbury Community Hospital in Sunbury, Pennsylvania, until retiring in 2000.

Cottrell was a member of the American Medical Association, the Eastern Orthopedic Association, the Pennsylvania Orthopedic Society, and the Pennsylvania Medical Association. He was a fellow of the American College of Surgeons, and the College of Physicians of Philadelphia and American Academy of Orthopedic Surgeons.

John E. Davis

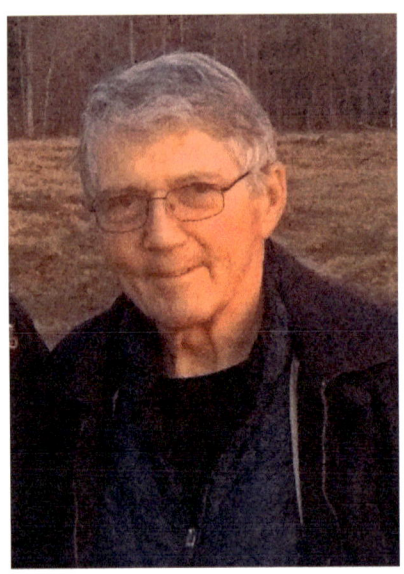

Born:	1943
Died:	2022
Years Active:	30+
Location:	North Carolina
Role(s):	Founder Mid-Carolina Orthopedics, pioneer orthopedic surgeon

Orthopedic surgeon John E. Davis, M.D., founded Mid-Carolina Orthopedics in North Carolina.

Dr. Davis was born in Youngstown, Ohio where he attended Boardman High School and played varsity football and golf.

After graduating in 1960, he attended Colgate University in Hamilton, New York and played football, lacrosse and was a member of Phi Delta Theta fraternity. He then went on to earn his medical degree in 1968 from Columbia University College of Physicians and Surgeons.

Following his internship at Grady Memorial Hospital in Atlanta, Georgia, Davis joined the U.S. Navy and served as a physician in Vietnam. After his tour in country, he continued his service at the Naval Hospital in Oakland, California.

Dr. Davis was honorably discharged from the Navy in June 1971 at the rank of lieutenant and went on to complete a four-year residency in orthopedics in Chattanooga, Tennessee.

In the early 1980s, Davis founded Mid-Carolina Orthopedics where he served patients in Tryon and Rutherfordton, North Carolina for over 30 years. Dr. Davis was a member of the Eastern Orthopedic Association, the Southern Orthopedic Association, and the North American Spine Society.

Leo De Souza

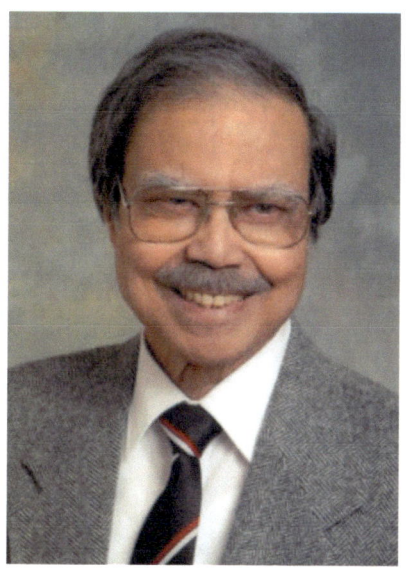

Born:	1927
Died:	2016
Years Active:	35+
Location:	Minnesota
Role(s):	Winner of the Life Time Achievement award from Hennepin County Medical Center, pioneering orthopedic surgeon

Leo de Souza, M.D., was born in Tanzania and went on to survive—and then escape—life under the Ugandan regime of Idi Amin. Dr. de Souza served patients at the Hennepin County Medical Center (HCMC) and the University of Minnesota.

Dr. de Souza received his medical training in India and Great Britain, and in 1961 was made a fellow of the Royal College of Surgeons, Edinburgh. After the military coup in Uganda Dr. de Souza and his family fled to Minnesota in 1971. He went to Toronto for re-certification, where he was made a Fellow of the Royal College of Surgeons of Canada. In November 2013, HCMC presented him with the Lifetime Achievement Award.

In his 70s, Dr. de Souza studied creative writing at Hamline University, earning Best Non-Fiction of the Year Award for 2002.

Richard Kyle, M.D., a past president of the American Academy of Orthopaedic Surgeons, did his residency under Dr. de Souza. "Leo was known for taking care of the less fortunate," remembers Kyle, "several years back he approached me and asked if I could operate on a Ugandan priest. I immediately agreed and now that priest is back in Africa ministering to people who don't have many resources."

"He did a lot of important clinical research in spine and foot and ankle. But I think his most significant contribution was the thousands of lectures he did for other physicians. He was named teacher of the year by residents and went to extraordinary lengths to continue helping students learn. When he was too ill to get out of bed, he phoned me and asked if he could teach residents and fellows via Skype. And that was just fine with me."

Jeffrey Thomas DeHaan

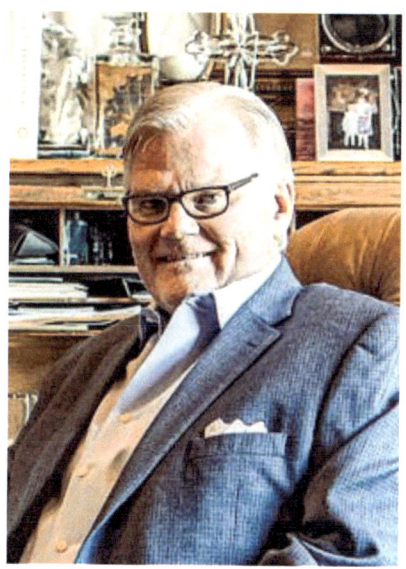

Born:	1956
Died:	2022
Years Active:	36+
Location:	Texarkana, TX
Role(s):	Pioneer Orthopedic Surgeon

Jeffrey Thomas DeHaan was born shortly after Charnley had his large joint arthroplasty 'eureka' moment. When Dr. DeHaan started his medical practice in Texarkana, Texas, and the surrounding communities, he was one of the first surgeons to perform that hip and knee arthroplasty. He served his community for more than 36 years,

Dr. DeHaan practiced at the Collom & Carney Clinic in Texarkana until he retired.

DeHaan received his medical degree from the University of Iowa Medical School. He went on to do his residency at The University of Texas in San Antonio from 1981 to 1986. He also did a fellowship in Switzerland.

DeHaan was born on July 7, 1955, and grew up in Orange City, Iowa. He attended Northwestern College in Orange City and there he played football and golf. His golf team won the College National Golf Championship and was inducted into Northwestern's golf hall of fame.

Robert Leonard Diaz

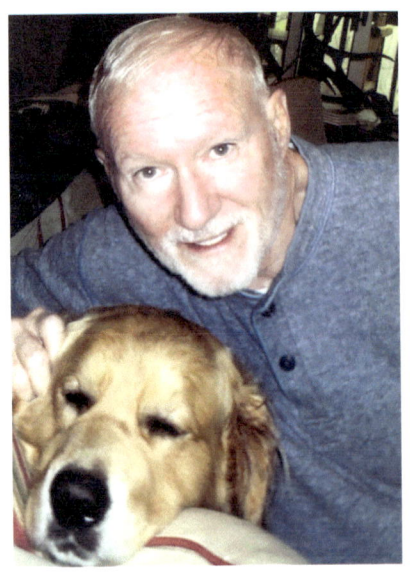

Born:	1936
Died:	2022
Years Active:	61
Location:	Jupiter, FL
Role(s):	Co-founder of Palm Beach Orthopedic Institute and Pioneer Orthopedic Surgeon

Robert Leonard Diaz was in practice for 61 years, was a co-founder of the Palm Beach Orthopedic Institute and one of the first orthopedic surgeons to offer joint arthroplasty in Southern Florida,

In addition to helping found the Palm Beach Orthopedic Institute, Dr. Diaz was also instrumental in the opening of the Jupiter Medical Center in Jupiter, Florida.

Dr. Diaz was one of the first doctors to perform total hip arthroplasty at St. Mary's Hospital.

Dr. Diaz was in practice for 61 years and became a nationally recognized opinion leader and expert in the practice of treating hip and knee osteoarthritis and hip and knee arthroplasty.

Diaz was born on April 19, 1936, in Brooklyn, New York, to Leonard Manuel Diaz and Doris Marshall Diaz. His family eventually settled in Baldwin, New York, on Long Island where he attended Baldwin High School. He graduated from Muhlenberg College in Allentown, Pennsylvania, and earned his medical degree from Hahnemann Medical School in Philadelphia.

He then went on to the world famous Hospital for Special Surgery in Manhattan for his orthopedic training. Before starting private practice as an orthopedic surgeon, he served two years in the U.S. Army.

William "Lonnie" Dillon

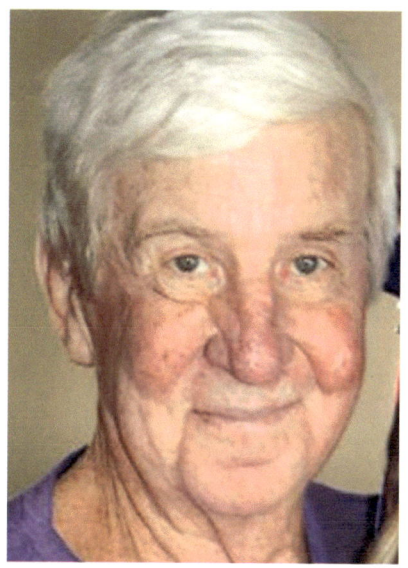

Born:	1945
Died:	2021
Years Active:	40+
Location:	Southeast Kansas
Role(s):	Pioneer Orthopedic Surgeon

William "Lonnie" Dillon, M.D., a pioneer orthopedic surgeon was one of the first surgeons to offer joint arthroplasty in Southeast Kansas and served patients for more than 40 years.

Dr. Dillon practiced his craft of orthopedic surgery and sports medicine at the Labette County Medical Center in Parsons, Kansas and at the Neosho Memorial Regional Medical Center in Chanute.

"Dr. Dillon served the patients of southeast Kansas with dignity, honor and an unmatched commitment to developing a nationally ranked orthopedic program" said Labette Health President and CEO Brian Williams.

Dillon's Southeast Kansas Orthopedic Clinic earned national recognition for its expertise and ability to bring the latest techniques to the entire southeast Kansas region. One of Dillon's colleagues, Dr. Kevin Mosier said, "If it wasn't for Dr. Dillon, there wouldn't be orthopedic surgery care here in Parsons as we know it today. He brought advanced orthopedic care here and put Parsons on the map as a center of excellence for bone and joint surgery here in Southeast Kansas. He was just an incredible, skilled, talented surgeon."

Dillon was born March 28, 1945, in Burr Oak, Kansas—a town of about 170 people near the Nebraska border and roughly 240 miles due west of Kansas City, Kansas. Dr. Dillon earned his bachelor's degree from Kansas State University and then graduated in 1971 with a Doctorate in Medicine from the University of Kansas Medical School.

With a degree in medicine, Dr. Dillion moved from his beloved Kansas to, first, Biloxi, Mississippi and then Anchorage, Alaska, where he served two residencies.

He then entered the U.S. Air Force and served as an orthopedic surgeon 1976 and 1980, earning the Meritorious Service Medal.

John Elliot

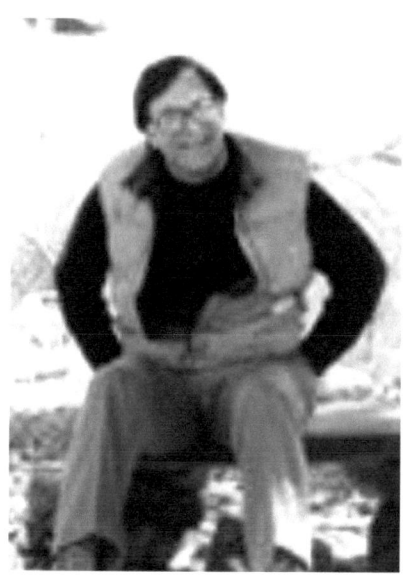

Born:	1933
Died:	2021
Years Active:	60+
Location:	Rhode Island and Connecticut
Role(s):	Chief of Staff and Surgery at Westerly Hospital. Assistant Clinical Professor of Orthopedics Yale University.

John Elliot, M.D., was a physician and orthopedic surgeon for more than 60 years. He served as Chief of Staff and Surgery at Westerly Hospital in Rhode Island and Assistant Clinical Professor of Orthopedics at Yale University.

John Elliott was born to an Italian immigrant family as Amerigo John Eleuteri on April 3, 1933.

A child of the Great Depression, Elliot's parents chose to have only one child so as to pour all resources into his education and future. His father Americus (Mike) and mother Theresa envisioned a bright future for their son, with Theresa telling Elliot from childhood that he would be a surgeon and working hard to provide piano lessons "to strengthen his hands."

Elliot was, in fact, valedictorian at Trenton High School, where he gave a passionate and well-received speech critiquing McCarthyism.

Rare for a public school student, Elliot subsequently attended Princeton University, where he bonded with friends at Phi Beta Kappa and graduated with a pre-med degree in 1955.

He then attended medical school at Columbia College of Physicians and Surgeons. Elliot graduated with the class of 1959 and entered into a surgery internship at Johns Hopkins Hospital from 1960-1961, followed by an ortho residency at Yale University from 1961-1964.

He chose to change his last name to Elliot during his medical residency because when called over the loudspeaker, the attendants often said "Elliot" rather than

"Eleuteri," either from an inability or an unwillingness to articulate his actual surname.

Elliot was both a gifted ortho surgeon and diagnostician. He often accepted barter as payment, filling his family home with soups, wines, baked goods and even a patient-constructed dock.

Elliot became Chief of Staff as well as Chief of Surgery at Westerly Hospital. He was also at one time an Assistant Clinical Professor of Orthopedics at Yale University.

Elliot attended Cambridge College in the UK in the early 1980s to study arthroscopy, then brought his learning to the Westerly Community. In 1986, he was a visiting professor at West China Medical University in Chengdu. He was, in fact, named Professor Emeritus by West China Medical University in 2020.

Clint Devin

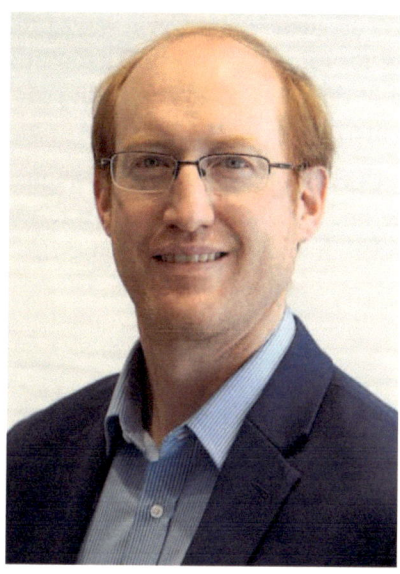

Dr. Clint Devin was head of spine trauma at Vanderbilt University in Nashville, Tennessee, and an adjunct associate professor of orthopedic surgery and neurosurgery at Vanderbilt University Medical Center before entering private practice as a spine surgeon at the Steamboat Orthopaedic and Spine Institute (SOSI) in Colorado.

Dr. Devin was instrumental in creating two spine surgery outcome registries and authored or co-authored 169 peer-reviewed publications.

Devin tracked patient outcomes originally through a database that started in 2009 at Vanderbilt and then through the American Spine Registry via the American Academy of Orthopaedic Surgeons.

"Dr. Devin was a national leader in developing and maintaining patient outcome databases in spine surgery in his efforts to deliver ethical spine care and improve patient outcomes," said SOSI Physician Assistant Jessica Nyquist. "He believed in holding surgeons accountable and was devoted to progressing and bettering spine care."

Dr. Devin received his medical degree at Vanderbilt University and completed his orthopedic residency at Vanderbilt University Medical Center in Nashville. He also completed a complex spinal-reconstruction fellowship at the University of Pittsburgh Medical Center.

He performed more than 5,500 spine surgeries of all levels of complexity over his surgical career. His philosophy was to provide the least invasive treatment possible that would still allow patients to return to doing what they loved.

Born:	1975
Died:	2021
Years Active:	20
Location:	Colorado
Role(s):	Head of Spine Trauma Vanderbilt University, Associate Professor of Orthopedic Surgery and Neurosurgery Vanderbilt.

Dr. Devin died when his plane crashed at the top of Emerald Mountain in northern Colorado while flying into Steamboat from Cody, Wyoming. He was the pilot and the only person on the plane.

Devin, 46 years old, was remembered by his colleagues: "Clint Devin was a brilliant spine surgeon who helped many to move forward in their journey towards healing. Dr. Devin was a driver in the creation of the new Steamboat Orthopedic and Spine Institute and Steamboat Surgical Center."

Prior to moving to Steamboat, Colorado, Dr. Devin was the head of spine trauma at Vanderbilt University in Nashville, Tennessee, and an adjunct associate professor of orthopedic surgery and neurosurgery at Vanderbilt University Medical Center.

Leonard D. Emond

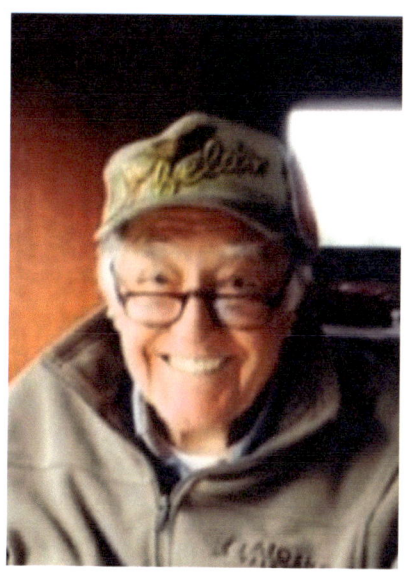

Born:	1929
Died:	2022
Years Active:	20+
Location:	Manchester, NH
Role(s):	Founding member and past president of the American Academy of Disability Evaluating Physicians, pioneering orthopedic surgeon and opera singer

Leonard D. Emond was a founding member and past president of the American Academy of Disability Evaluating Physicians, orthopedic surgeon and opera singer.

Dr. Emond brought joint arthroplasty to patients in the Manchester, New Hampshire region was affiliated with Manchester Veterans Affairs Medical Center.

He served as a staff member at the Catholic Medical Center in Manchester, New Hampshire, from 1965 until his retirement.

Emond was born on August 20, 1928, in Greenville, New Hampshire. His parents were the late Charles D. and Albina Emond. He completed his Bachelor of Science at the University of New Hampshire in 1950 and then earned his medical degree from the University of Laval Faculty of Medicine in Quebec City, Canada, in 1956.

He completed an orthopedic surgery residency at Akron General Medical Center in Ohio and spent time practicing at Bradford Regional Medical Center in Bradford, Pennsylvania. He also did post graduate work at the University of Pennsylvania.

Emond was a member of multiple choruses in New Hampshire. His passion was singing opera. He also enjoyed mountain climbing and was a member of the Appalachian Mountain Club and the New Hampshire 4,000 Foot Club. He was one of the founding members of the Manhattan Hiking Club.

Timothy M. George

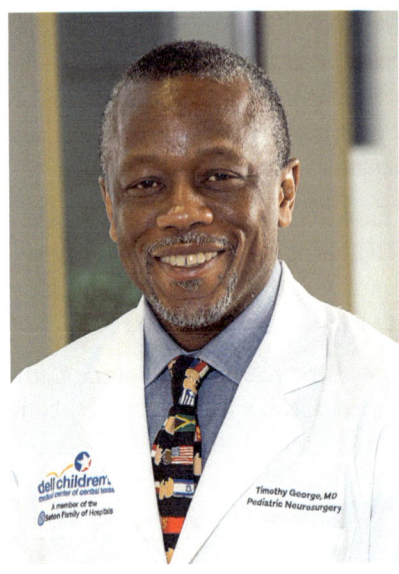

Born:	1960
Died:	2019
Years Active:	30+
Location:	Austin, TX
Role(s):	Chief of Pediatric Neurosurgery, President Dell Children's Medical Group

Dr. Timothy M. George was Chief of Pediatric Neurosurgery, President of Dell Children's Medical Group, mentor to dozens of his neurosurgery colleagues and prolific researcher in the areas of Chiari malformation, cranial nerve stimulation for pediatric epilepsy, genomics of neural tube defects, and other current neurosurgery topics.

The youngest of three children, Dr. George was born in Brooklyn, New York, in 1960 to Carey and Gracie George. Amazingly, he knew at age four, after watching an open heart surgery on television, that he wanted to grow up to be a surgeon. His family remembers the young Tim George in much the same way his patients would later remember him — calm, cool, collected and intensely interested in other people.

In his youth he was a camp counselor for children with disabilities and that, eventually, would lead him into a career in pediatrics. He also worked alongside his father as an apprentice plumber.

He was a proud graduate of Long Island Lutheran High School in Brookville, New York, where he not only excelled scholastically but was the starting point guard on the championship varsity basketball team.

Between high school and NYU med school, Tim attended Columbia University and, in his spare time, played plenty of round ball, DJ'd around New York City, developed his lifelong passion for sports cars and formed TIMARI.

Dr. George completed his residency in neurosurgery at Yale University and stayed to continue his neurosurgical training. He added subspecialty training in pediatric neurosurgery at Northwestern University.

In 1996 he moved to Duke University to join the neurosurgery faculty. Dr. George was soon invited to join the Duke faculty as an Associate Professor with Tenure. His area of specialty was pediatric congenital abnormalities and tumors.

In 2006 Dr. George accepted the position of professor for the Department of Neurology and the medical director of the Pediatric Neurosurgery Center of Central Texas at Dell Children's Medical Center in Austin, Texas.

Here he was able to build on his passion for pediatric neurosurgery, train and mentor the next generation of neurosurgeons and continue his research in genomics and surgical outcomes of Chiari malformation, cranial nerve stimulation for pediatric epilepsy, genomics of neural tube defects, and molecular and cellular mechanisms and abnormal development of the spinal cord.

He was a member of the American Society of Pediatric Neurosurgeons, the Congress of Neurological Surgeons, the American Academy of Pediatrics, the Sigma Pi Phi fraternity, the Austin Black Physicians Association and other scientific societies and organizations.

Tim George was also an accomplished, professional race car driver.

According to his fellow sportscar drivers, he was one of the most popular drivers on the International Motor Sports Association (IMSA) paddock, having competed in the likes of the Mazda Prototype Challenge, FARA, and IMSA lights series. Tim competed nationally with the Sports Car Club of America and achieved podium finishes in both his Mazda MX5 racecar and his Pro Formula Mazda.

His success and passion for the sport earned him his FIA International Competition License (Federation Internationale de l'Automobile) to compete with the International Motor Sports Association in his first prototype racecar, the Elan DP02.

He competed successfully as a pro driver at Road Atlanta, Watkins Glen in New York, Homestead Raceway in Florida and at Sebring International Raceway as well as many other raceways across the country.

Dr. George died unexpectedly on November 10, 2019, while participating in the four-hour Michelin IMSA SportsCar Encore at Sebring International Raceway.

Dr. George was driving a No. 2 Ansa Motorsports LLC prototype race car when he began experiencing severe medical problems. He was able to drive the car onto the pit lane. Despite the best efforts of track medical personnel and later emergency room staff at the closest Sebring hospital, Tim George's extraordinary life came to a premature end.

Larry Khoo, M.D., magna cum laude graduate from Yale Medical School and prolific neurosurgeon and investigator with over 60 peer reviewed journal articles,

10 patents, 60 book chapters, 2 full books, and 400 scientific presentations under his belt said this about his mentor, Dr. Tim George: "Dr. Tim George was my chief resident when I was a Yale Medical Student. I am a neurosurgeon now in large part due to his mentorship and friendship."

Walter T. Gilsdorf

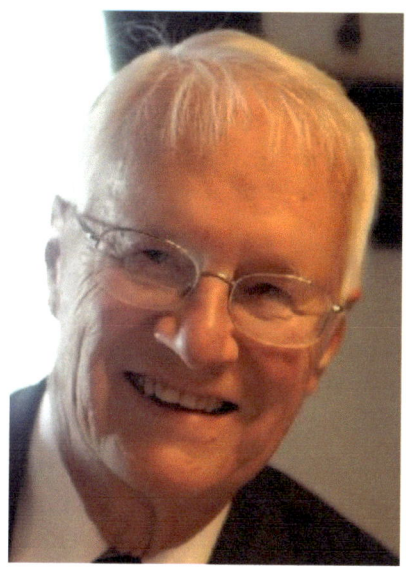

Born:	1934
Died:	2022
Years Active:	35+
Location:	Lafayette, NY
Role(s):	Pioneering Orthopedic Surgeon and Member of the New York State Board of Professional Medical Conduct

Walter T. Gilsdorf, from Lafayette, New York, was a member of the New York State Board for Professional Medical Conduct.

Gilsdorf, who was born on April 10, 1934, graduated from Harvard Medical School in 1959, did a surgical residency at the University of Iowa Hospitals and Clinics between 1960 and 1962 and also at SUNY Upstate Medical University in 1965.

Dr. Gilsdorf spent the majority of his career serving his community in Lafayette, New York. In addition to his orthopedic practice, Dr. Gilsdorf also served on Lafayette, New York's School Board and was a member of the Lafayette Optimist Club whose mission is to serve their community and to make a difference to every person they meet.

Those closest to him said that Dr. Gilsdorf's approach to life could be summed up as: "work hard, play hard, learn hard and revel in life's challenges and joys." He put everything he had into everything he did.

Pau Golano

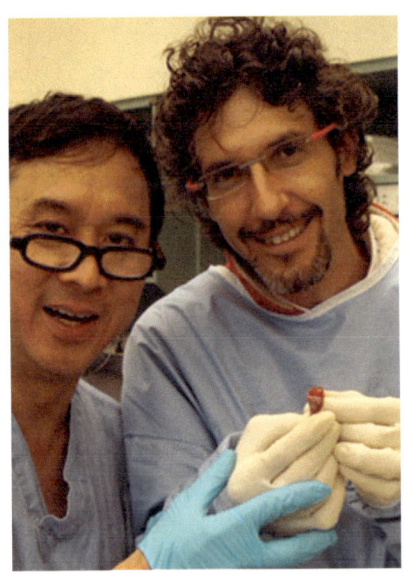

Born:	1965
Died:	2014
Years Active:	20+
Location:	Barcelona, Spain
Role(s):	Professor of Pathology and Experimental Therapeutics, University of Barcelona, Adjunct Faculty University of Pittsburgh Medical Center

Pau Golanó was the Professor of Pathology and Experimental Therapeutics at the University of Barcelona, an adjunct member of the University of Pittsburgh Medical Center faculty and one of best anatomists in the world.

In 2012 he was given the ESSKA award for service as the Most Dedicated Individual Member at the 16th Congress in 2012 in Geneva and won KSSTA Best Paper Award for "Anatomy of the Ankle Ligaments: a Pictorial Essay."

Niek van Dijk, president of the ESSKA Ankle & Foot Associates said of Professor Golanó, "...His exceptional anatomical dissection skills and passion for education was quickly recognized by the orthopaedic surgeons surrounding him. And it did not take long before his skills were recognized worldwide, and he became the leading expert on orthopaedic anatomy of the last decade."

"He devoted his career and life to the education of orthopaedic surgeons, making them better doctors by teaching anatomy in the finest details...Over the years he has written many inspiring papers on orthopaedic surgical anatomy."

"Once every two years we organized in Barcelona a dissection course for all the residents of our Department. We practiced all the open surgical approaches. Pau Golanó was our teacher. But Pau was a teacher for all orthopaedic surgeons."

From the European Society of Sports Traumatology, Knee Surgery, and Arthroscopy, "Pau Golanó was a very talented anatomist who helped shape and advance orthopaedic surgery. He was considered by many to be the best musculoskeletal anatomist in the world."

Freddie Fu, M.D., David Silver Professor and Chairman of the Department of Orthopaedic Surgery, University of Pittsburgh School of Medicine, said, "Pau was well known for his irreplaceable skills to anatomical dissection and passion for education. After visiting in the summer of 2008, he continued to collaborate with our department and provided musculoskeletal anatomy lectures to our residents, fellows, and medical students."

Todd Graham

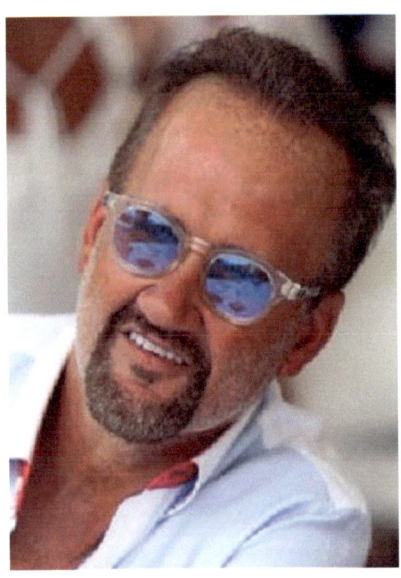

For more than 30 years, Dr. Todd Graham has served orthopedic patients in the northern Indiana region.

Dr. Graham began his career as a solo practitioner and successfully operated his private practice for 22 years. He then went on to become a partner at South Bend Orthopedics, where he was elected a member of the executive committee.

Over the course of three decades, Dr. Graham became ingrained in the greater South Bend region's medical and philanthropic communities. He volunteered with the University of Notre Dame as a consultant for its athletics program.

Dr. Graham was born on October 30, 1960 in Athens, Illinois, to Jean and Jack Graham. He went on to graduate from the University of Illinois, Champaign-Urbana and then Northwestern University School of Medicine. He was double board certified in both Physical Medicine & Rehabilitation and Pain Medicine. After medical school, he went to South Bend, Indiana.

On July 26, 2017, Dr. Graham had an appointment with a new patient and her husband at his South Bend Orthopedics office. At the appointment, the patient described her symptoms and then asked Dr. Graham to prescribe opioids. Dr. Graham informed the couple that, even though she suffered from pain, he could not prescribe opioids for her.

Two hours later, unbeknownst to the wife, the husband returned to the medical complex.

The husband confronted Dr. Graham in the parking lot of the St. Joseph Rehabilitation Institute next door to the orthopedic center. According to the *South*

Born:	1960
Died:	2017
Years Active:	45+
Location:	Northern Indiana
Role(s):	Pioneering orthopedic surgeon and partner in South Bend Orthopedics

Bend Tribune, the husband told two witnesses to leave and then shot Dr. Graham twice in the head.

He then went to a friend's house and shot and killed himself.

His son, Travis Graham, M.D., issued a statement saying his father inspired him to pursue his own career in medicine.

"My father's passion for medicine inspired me to follow his footsteps," Travis Graham said. "I had less than a year to finish my residency program before joining him as a doctor in South Bend. Even though we won't get to practice at the same time now, I hope I can be the kind of doctor he would be proud of."

Frank Benton Gray

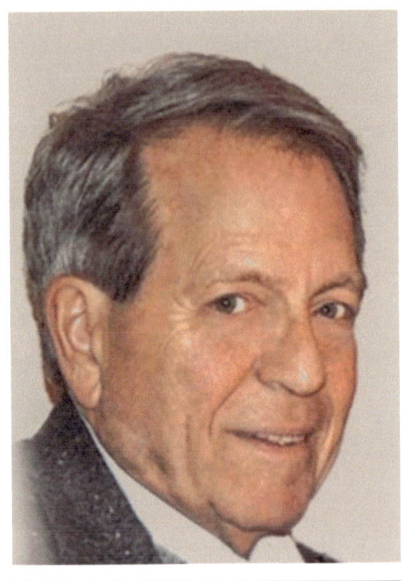

Frank Benton Gray, M.D., is the co-founder of the Society for Arthritic Joint Surgery and over the 34 year course of his exceptional career, he treated orthopedic patients in the Knoxville, Tennessee region --and then volunteered at Knoxville's InterFaith Health Clinic which serves 24,000 low income, uninsured patients for another 17 years.

Dr. Gray is a 1969 graduate of the University of North Carolina School of Medicine. While attending medical school he co-founded the Student Health Action Coalition. A first in the country, the student-run clinic recently celebrated its 50th anniversary.

Dr. Gray received his surgical training at Duke University Medical Center and then volunteered for service in the U.S. Navy before returning to Duke for his residency in orthopedic surgery. In 1977, he moved with his family to Knoxville and joined the Knoxville Orthopedic Clinic. He specialized in total hip and total knee replacement.

In 1983, Dr. Gray co-founded the Society for Arthritic Joint Surgery. During his career, he was active in several medical and orthopedic societies. His interests included orthopedic product development and he obtained several patents. Listed among the Best Doctors in America, Dr. Gray retired in 2000. He continued to serve patients as an InterFaith Health Clinic volunteer physician until 2017.

Born:	1942
Died:	2020
Years Active:	50+ (includes 17 volunteer yrs.)
Location:	Knoxville, TN
Role(s):	Co-founder of the Society for Arthritic Joint Surgery, co-founder of the Student Health Action Coalition and 17 years volunteering at InterFaith Health Clinic in Knoxville

Dr. Gray, who was born in 1942 in Durham, North Carolina, had always had a passion for playing classical music on the piano. His major at Duke University was piano with a pre-med focus.

For more than 40 years, Dr. Gray served as a board member of the Knoxville Symphony Orchestra. During retirement he played on his Steinway model D concert grand piano for at least an hour each day.

Eugene "Gene" Frank Gulish

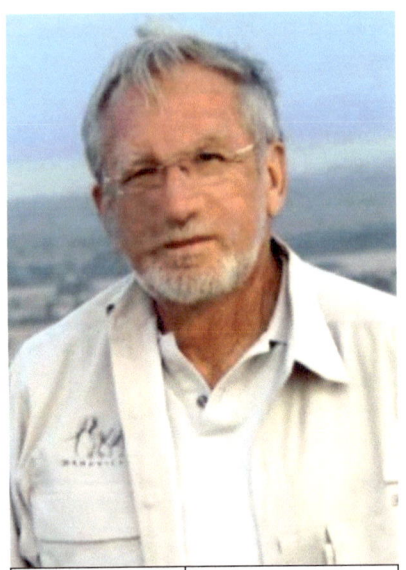

Born:	1937
Died:	2022
Years Active:	42
Location:	Sonoma County, CA and Northwestern TN
Role(s):	Pioneering orthopedic surgeon, Sonoma County, California and Paris, Tennesee

Dr. Eugene "Gene" Frank Gulish, entered the practice of orthopedics when joint arthroplasty was still in its inaugural decade. He brought large joint arthroplasty to Sonoma County, California, specifically the small community of Sebastopol.

After 22 years in wine country, Dr. Gulish and his wife moved to Paris, Tennessee, an equally small town (about 10,000 residents) in northwestern Tennessee, just south of the Kentucky border. Dr. Gulish would serve as that regions primary orthopedic surgeon for another 20 years.

Dr. Gulish served his country as an Army orthopedic surgeon at Fort Polk and later, in country, in Vietnam. Later in his professional life, Dr. Gulish participated in several volunteer surgical trips to Africa.

Gulish was born on January 10, 1937, in Curtice, Ohio. He grew up on a small farm and graduated from Clay High School in 1955. He was the first person in his family to graduate from high school.

He attended the University of Michigan and then earned his medical degree from The Ohio State University. He completed his residency at Los Angeles County General Hospital.

After his residency he volunteered for the U.S. Army and received the Army Commendation Medal in 1971.

After discharge, he set up his orthopedic practice in Sebastopol, California.

He also started farming and keeping bees.

In 1994, he was recruited by Henry County Medical Center in Paris, Tennessee. When he and his family visited the area, they fell in love with the community and made the move. He was the primary orthopedic surgeon in that region of Tennesee for over 20 years.

After retiring, he worked another two years in McKenzie and Huntingdon, Tennessee and, of course, maintained his farm and kept his bees.

Armen Charles Haig

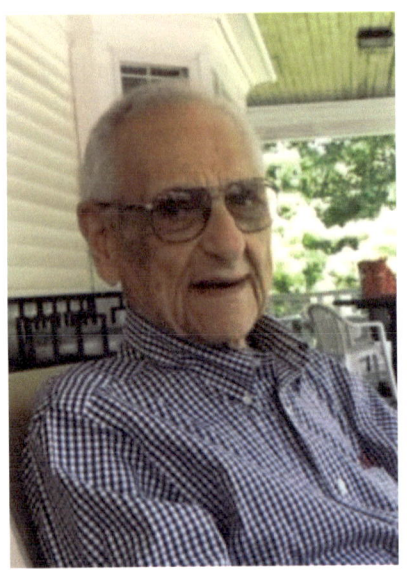

Born:	1932
Died:	2022
Years Active:	50+
Location:	Bronxville, NY
Role(s):	Pioneering Orthopedic Surgeon, Chief of Staff and Chief of Orthopedics, Lawrence Hospital, Bronxville, NY, Clinical Professor of Surgery, Columbia University, New York City.

Armen Charles Haig, M.D., was the former chief of staff and orthopedics at Lawrence Hospital in Bronxville, New York.

As an orthopedic surgeon, he served the Westchester County, New York, for more than 50 years. During his career at Lawrence Hospital, Dr. Haig was chief of orthopedics for two terms and chief of staff for another two. He also was assistant clinical professor of orthopedic surgery at Columbia Presbyterian in New York City.

It was always his childhood dream to become a surgeon. He loved what he did so much, he often spent holidays, even Christmas day, at the hospital visiting patients, even when he wasn't on call.

Haig was born on March 9, 1932, in New York City, where he attended Stuyvesant High School. He then earned his bachelor's degree from Columbia College in Manhattan. He received medical degree at Yale University School of Medicine in 1956. Dr. Haig served as an active duty U.S. Air Force Captain for two years and then in the Air Force Reserve eight years.

William H.B. Howard

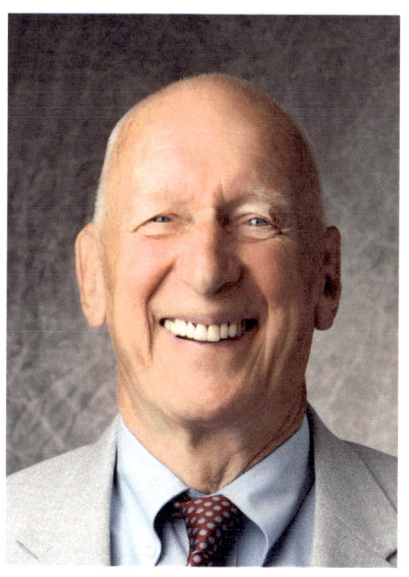

Born:	1935
Died:	2016
Years Active:	40+
Location:	Baltimore, MD
Role(s):	Pioneering Sport Medicine Orthopedist, Medical Director and co-founder Medstar Union Memorial Sports Medicine Clinic

William H.B. Howard, M.D. was the longtime medical director and co-founder of MedStar Union Memorial's Sports Medicine Clinic.

Dr. Howard entered the world at Union Memorial Hospital, and several years later began his education in a one-room schoolhouse. He then attended Duke University and followed that up with a bachelor's degree from the Johns Hopkins University. He was a 1963 graduate of the University of Maryland School of Medicine.

He did his residency in general surgery and orthopedics at Harrisburg Hospital in Pennsylvania and returned to Baltimore, where he ran the emergency room at what is now MedStar Union Memorial Hospital (UMH).

Convinced of the profound need for a disciplined, scientific orthopedic treatment for athletes, Dr. Howard worked with Drs. Joe Martire, a radiologist, and Roger Michael, then chief of orthopedics, to open a sports medicine clinic, one of the first in the United States, in 1979.

Stuart B. Bell, M.D., vice president, Medical Affairs and CMO of MedStar Union Memorial Hospital, said of Dr. Howard; "Dr. Howard was the face of UMH for at least 40 years, an iconic figure. He founded the critical program in UMH development, our Sports Medicine program, based on an idea he had (and he had many) derived from his work running our Emergency Department, where he would see athletes from Memorial stadium, down the street, for sports injuries. Our sports medicine programs, those of MedStar, and to some extent, our successful orthopaedic programs, are a direct result of his founding efforts."

"He taught many of our clinicians, students, nurses, doctors, and also the public at large in his media persona. He reached many in his time here."

Joseph A. Izzi Sr

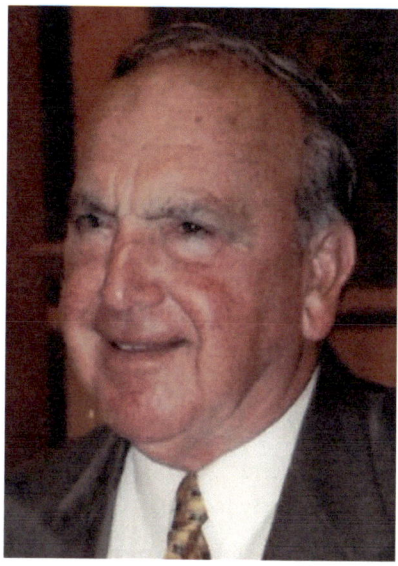

Born:	1935
Died:	2022
Years Active:	45
Location:	Providence, RI
Role(s):	Pioneer Joint Arthroplasty Surgeon

Joseph A. Izzi, Sr., M.D., Vietnam veteran and Rhode Island-based orthopedic surgeon, began his orthopedic practice when arthroplasty was still a new and developing technique for treating severe joint arthritis.

Dr. Izzi, one of the first joint arthroplasty surgeons in the Providence and North Providence, Rhode Island area, served his patients for 45 years.

His was an active and key member of the Providence Medical Society, Rhode Island Orthopaedic Society, American College of Surgeons, International College of Surgeons, The American Academy of Orthopaedics Surgeons, University of Bologna Alumni Association, Eastern Orthopaedic Society and the Irish American Orthopaedic Society, a professional organization for orthopedic surgeons who are Irish, of Irish descent, or have trained in an Irish University.

Dr. Izzi Sr. was born on February 12, 1935, to Carolyn and Roger Izzi. He attended La Salle Academy in Providence, Rhode Island, and then earned his bachelor's degree from Providence College.

Dr. Izzi Sr. received his medical degree from The University of Bologna Medical School in Italy and then came home for his internship and orthopedic residency at Rhode Island Hospital.

He then took his medical training and served his country in the Vietnam war as a Lt. Commander in the U.S. Navy. Among his postings was Da Nang, during the infamous and tragic Tet Offensive.

Jesse George Jackson

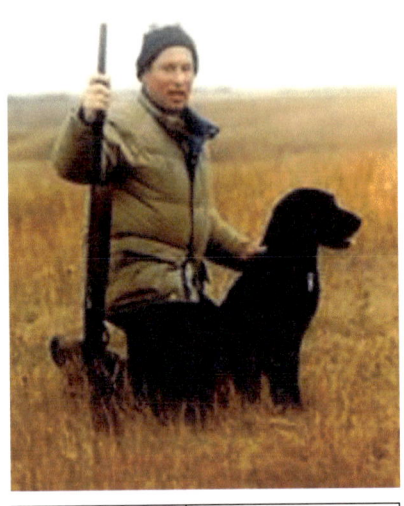

Born:	1935
Died:	2015
Years Active:	40+
Location:	Western United States
Role(s):	One of the first orthopedic product distributors, "Godfather" of orthopedics and the largest Zimmer distributor in the U.S.

Jesse George Jackson was one of the earliest orthopedic product distributors in the modern era and the person who was described by one friend as the "Godfather" of orthopedics in the West.

In addition to building the distribution, training and support infrastructure for modern orthopedic products and services in the western states, Jackson also co-invented (with Craig Shelling) a novel cannulated bone screw in 2005 (patent # 7731738).

Longtime friends Rob and Tonya Behrens said of Jesse Jackson:

"Jesse George Jackson, a past CEO of OrthoPro and at one point, the largest Zimmer distributor in the U.S., was known as the Godfather of Orthopaedics in the West. Jesse personally changed the lives of thousands of young men and women and made them better. I am one of those men. He gave me an opportunity 29 years ago that changed the course of my life. His legacy will never be forgotten."

Radd Berrett remembers, of his friend, Jesse Jackson; "My job interview with Jesse was a four-day road trip through Idaho, Wyoming, and Montana. We hit every hospital, doctor, and fly-fishing spot on the map; and cleaned up at all of them. To this day, over 25 years later, I still live my life with his 'It's not about the destination—there isn't one. It's all a journey' approach to life."

"There was truly only one Jess Jackson," said Steve Phippen; "Jess was known for giving people chances. He gave me my first opportunity to break into an industry that I've loved from day one. It changed my life and the life of my family for the better."

"Mentoring was important to Jess, and he glowed brightest when speaking of the next young person he was bringing into the industry and how well they were doing. At a critical decision-making point in my career, Jess dropped everything and took four days to drive with me to Seattle from Salt Lake City to consult with another person in the industry. He only did this for my personal benefit; there was no way for Jess to benefit from this trip."

"I also want to note that he was a non-judgmental person. Jess circulated with people from every walk of life and background, and all were comfortable in his presence. You could be exactly who you are when with Jess Jackson."

Walter "Bill" Hughey King Jr.

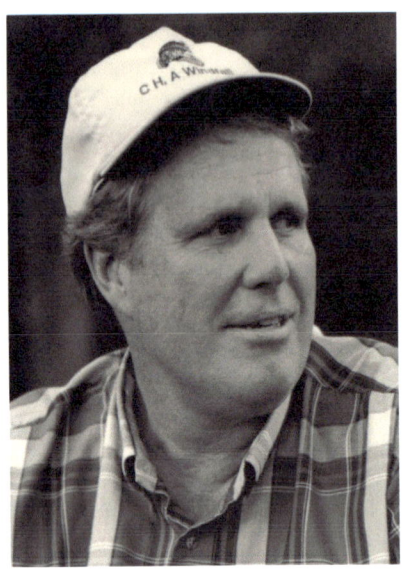

Born:	1942
Died:	2022
Years Active:	35+
Location:	Chattanooga, TN
Role(s):	Pioneer orthopedic surgeon, Assistant Professor of Medicine, University of Tennessee Chattanooga

Walter "Bill" Hughey King, Jr., M.D., was an orthopedic surgeon in Chattanooga, Tennessee, for over 35 years.

Dr. King served in many medical leadership roles over the years. He was an assistant professor of medicine at the University of Tennessee Chattanooga and volunteered at the Boehm Birth Defects Center for many years.

He gave back to the community in other ways too. He was a member of The Society of the Cincinnati, and a founding member of the Stones River Charter of the National Society of Sons of the American Revolution. He also served in the Army Reserves.

King was born to Sarah and Walter Hughey King, Sr. at St. Thomas Hospital in Nashville, Tennessee, on February 13, 1942. His early schooling was at Montgomery Bell Academy for junior high and Castle Heights Military Academy in Lebanon for high school. He attended Vanderbilt University but completed his bachelor's degree at Middle Tennessee State University.

He then earned his medical degree at the University of Tennessee Health Science Center Medical School and did his orthopedic surgery residency at Virginia Commonwealth University School of Medicine.

Petar Kokan

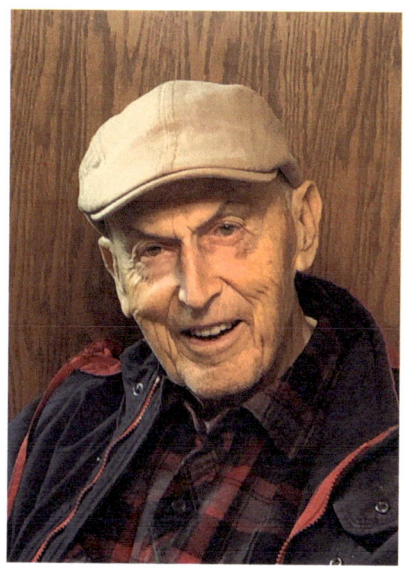

Petar Kokan, who was born in Croatia, later became a refugee and, then, for 30 years was a prominent orthopedic surgeon in Vancouver, Canada and one of the first large joint arthroplasty surgeons in British Columbia.

Kokan was born on July 9, 1930, and grew up in Split, Croatia. He was forced to flee the former Yugoslavia with his soon to be wife Nada a few years after graduating from the University of Zagreb medical school.

He completed a residency in general surgery in before moving to Canada in 1961. He lived and worked in Toronto, Victoria, and Nelson before ultimately settling full time in Vancouver in 1968.

Born:	1930
Died:	2022
Years Active:	39
Location:	Vancouver, Canada
Role(s):	Large joint arthroplasty pioneer

Kokan completed his residency in orthopedic surgery in Vancouver then practiced as an orthopedic surgeon at St. Paul's Hospital as well as Shaughnessy and Mount St. Joseph's Hospitals until he closed his medical practice in 2000.

Dr. Kokan continued to consult and assisting in the operating room for years after retiring.

"Petar was very proud to be a part of the Croatian community and the Catholic faith. During his lifetime he never complained, or feared anything, even when his health started finally catching up to his age. He remained humble, resilient, and a true gentleman for his entire life," his family said.

Alfred Kritter

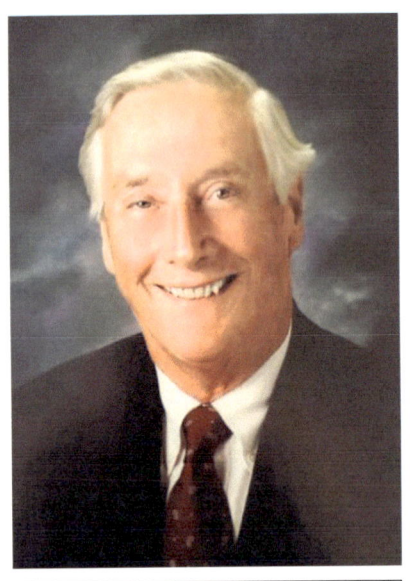

Born:	1929
Died:	2022
Years Active:	30+
Location:	Waukesha County, WI
Role(s):	Founder of Orthopaedic Associates of Wisconsin, Founder Juvenile Amputee and Congenital Limb Deficiency Center, Chief of Orthopedic Surgery Waukesha Memorial Hospital and clinical professor of Orthopedic Surgery at Medical College of Wisconsin.

Dr. Alfred Kritter was the first practicing orthopedic surgeon in Waukesha County, Wisconsin. His initial private practice is better known today as the Orthopaedic Associates of Wisconsin. He is also the founder of the Juvenile Amputee and Congenital Limb Deficiency Center at Children's Hospital of Wisconsin as well as the Milwaukee County General Hospital (now Froedtert) Adult Amputee Clinic.

During his long career, he was chief of orthopedic surgery at Waukesha Memorial Hospital, assistant clinical professor of orthopedic surgery at the Medical College of Wisconsin and held many local hospital affiliations.

Dr. Kritter published many articles in local, state, and international publications. In addition, he participated in the Doctors Without Borders program, where he traveled from Arizona to Mexico to donate his medical skills to desperately underserved communities in Mexico.

Born in Youngstown, Ohio on August 13, 1928, to the late Eugene and Helen Kritter, Dr. Kritter would later graduate from Marquette University and Marquette Medical School, where he also did his residency. He began his orthopedic practice in Waukesha, Wisconsin in 1960.

Alfred Kritter served active duty in the Korean War and then re-enlisted in the army as a field physician during the first Gulf War, retiring with the rank of colonel.

Seung "Sam" Chan Lee

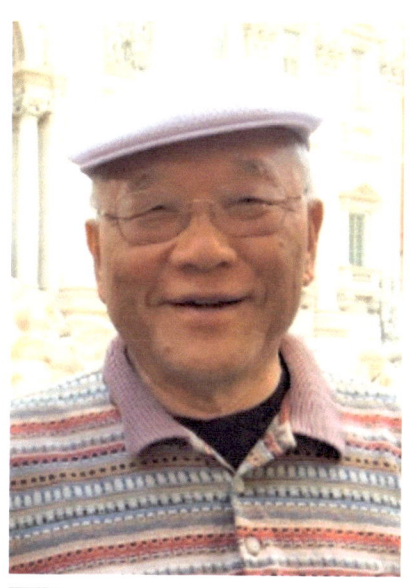

Seung "Sam" Chan Lee, M.D., 85, was an orthopedic surgeon and professor at the Catholic University of Korea during the formative years of modern orthopedics. He and his wife Pok Sil Song immigrated to the United States in the early 1970s.

They settled in Meadville, Pennsylvania, where Dr. Lee worked for almost 30 years at Meadville Medical Center. He was chief of anesthesiology and became an integral part of Meadville Medical community.

Lee was born in Korea on January 15, 1937. He graduated from the Catholic University of Korea in 1962 and served in the Korean navy during the Vietnam War before deciding to move to the United States.

Born:	1937
Died:	2022
Years Active:	
Location:	South Korea and Meadville, Pennsylvania
Role(s):	Large Joint Arthroplasty pioneer, Professor of orthopedic surgery at the Catholic University School of Medicine of Korea.

Dean Lorich

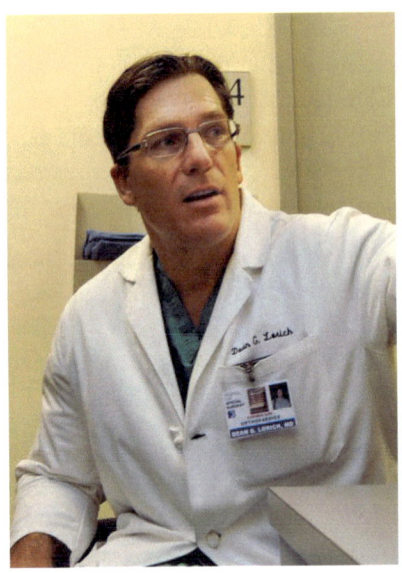

Born:	1963
Died:	2017
Years Active:	18
Location:	New York City
Role(s):	Associate Director Orthopedic Trauma Service, Hospital for Special Surgery, New York Presbyterian Hospital

Dean Lorich, M.D. was associate director of the Orthopedic Trauma Service at Hospital for Special Surgery (HSS) and director of the Orthopedic Trauma Service at New York Presbyterian Hospital.

One of a team of healthcare providers from HSS who rushed to aid the victims of the 2010 earthquake in Haiti, Dr. Lorich perform many surgeries and save lives. But he also ended up helping in a way that he likely didn't anticipate...he shone a light on shortcomings in the "giving" system.

He bravely exposed severe inadequacies on the part of the U.S. government and non-governmental organizations...and he wanted his colleagues to know the reality of providing aid in that disaster.

As Dr. Lorich—along with colleagues Drs. Soumitra Eachempati and David L. Helfet—wrote in a January 25, 2010, article that appeared on CNN, "Still, nobody with a clear plan is in charge, and care is chaotic at best. Doctors are coming into the country with no plan of what they are going to do, and nobody directing them how to do it. Surgeons who expect to show up and operate will be mistaken. Without a complement of support staff and supplies, they are of limited to no value."

Dr. Lorich earned his medical degree from the Perelman School of Medicine at the University of Pennsylvania and followed that with an orthopedic residency at the University of Pennsylvania Health System.

David Helfet, M.D., chief emeritus of the Orthopedic Trauma Service at HSS, said, "Dean was a superb, well-respected surgeon, teacher, colleague and friend to me and the entire Hospital for Special Surgery and New York-Presbyterian community. Throughout his 18-year career he impacted the lives of thousands of patients both near and far."

Bernard Allan Lublin

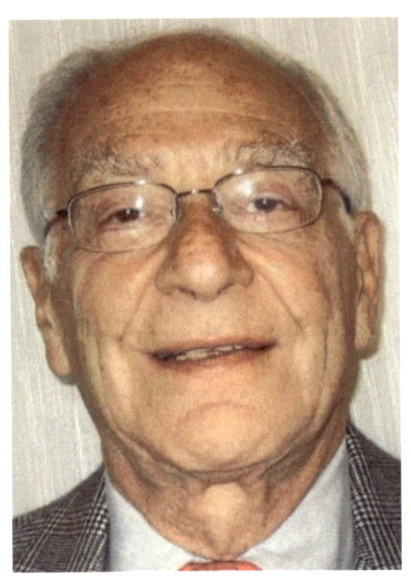

Born:	1937
Died:	2022
Years Active:	
Location:	
Role(s):	Founder of the Jewish Genetic Foundation, Changed how the medical community diagnoses and treats breast and ovarian oncologies, cancers which are able to metastasize into the musculoskeletal system.

Dr. Bernard Allan Lublin, an orthopedic surgeon, changed how chromosomal mutations, which appear at above average rates in women of Ashkenazi-Jewish decent, are incorporated into the diagnosis and treatment of those cancers, which are related, as well, to bone tumors.

Because of his remarkable work in this area, Dr. Lublin went on to establish the Jewish Genetic Foundation, which is now part of American Technion Society, and convinced the National Comprehensive Cancer Network to change their guidelines for the prophylactic treatment of these diseases.

He also convinced Myriad Genetics to develop and license pre-implantation genetic diagnosis for the first time.

Those who knew him best, his family and friends, said of Dr. Lublin, that "any mysterious medical symptom was a problem to be fully investigated, solved and addressed. Bernie always remembered the quote he first heard upon graduation from Yale, 'We'll all do well; may some do good.'"

Lublin was from Henrico, Virginia, and attended Yale University and New York University Medical School. He also served as a lieutenant in the U.S. Navy. In 1960, he moved to Richmond to complete an internship and residency in orthopedic surgery at Medical College of Virginia.

Dr. Lublin received the 2016 Jewish National Fund of Southwest Florida's Lifetime Achievement Award.

Dean Maar

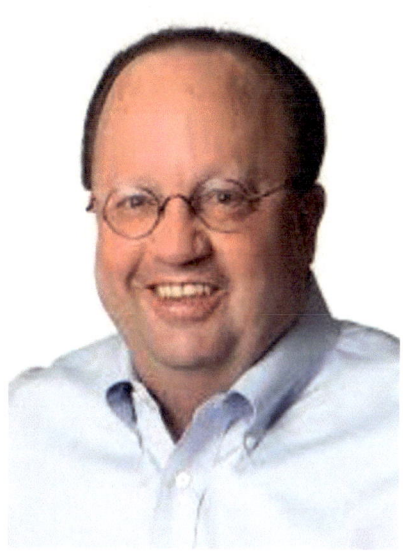

Born:	1958
Died:	2019
Years Active:	28
Location:	Indianapolis, IN
Role(s):	Board Member and Vice President of OrthoIndy. Instrumental in developing one of the leading trauma programs in the United States.

Dean Maar, M.D., was a largely unheralded leader in the orthopedic community, quietly leading his colleagues and Indiana community.

A board certified orthopedic surgeon, he practiced at one of the leading orthopedic institutions in the United States, OrthoIndy.

"Dr. Dean Maar has been a cornerstone of OrthoIndy as a previous board member and former Vice President and was instrumental to the development of our renowned trauma program. He brought integrity in all aspects of his patient care and contributions to the practice," said Tim Dicke, M.D., president and CEO of OrthoIndy.

Dr. Maar completed his undergraduate studies at DePauw University in Greencastle, graduating in 1981. He graduated from Indiana University School of Medicine in 1985 and completed an orthopedic residency at Indiana University School of Medicine in 1990.

He completed two fellowships in 1991: one in total hip and knee adult reconstructive surgery at Johns Hopkins University in Baltimore, Maryland, and another in Ilizarov Reconstruction at the University of Maryland in Baltimore.

Dr. Maar had manuscripts published in *Orthopedics*, *The Journal of Bone and Joint Surgery*, *The Journal of Arthroplasty* and other medical periodicals. He has presented on national and international levels and served as the assistant editor for *The Journal of Arthroplasty* from 1991 to 1999.

Indianapolis Monthly named him as a "Top Doctors" from 2014 - 2019.

With more than 70 orthopedic specialists and 11 locations, OrthoIndy is the largest physician-owned, full-service orthopedic practice in the Midwest, and one of the largest in the country.

Dean Maar, while preparing to host a large, extended family Thanksgiving dinner in 2019, was confronted in his home by armed attackers and, sacrificed his life to save his wife and family.

Dr. Maar made a quick decision under intense pressure and with little time for reflection to save lives and limbs – as he had done for decades as a trauma surgeon, noted those who knew him best.

Investigators believe this was an attempted robbery. They also said a small fire appeared to be intentionally set inside the home but was quickly put out by first responders.

Theodore Maravich

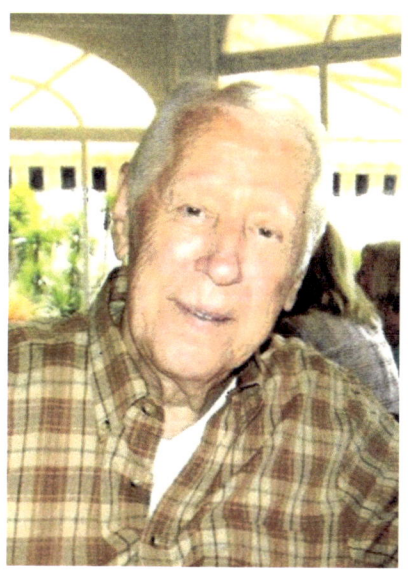

Theodore Maravich, M.D., was one of the first orthopedic surgeons specializing in large joint arthroplasty in southern California. Dr. Maravich was also associate clinical professor in orthopedics at the University of California at Irvine.

Dr. Maravich was a fellow of the American Academy of Orthopedic.

He was born in Aliquippa, Pennsylvania on December 3, 1931, to Dmitar and Boja Maravich. He was one of six children.

Dr. Maravich served in the United Dates Army straight out of high school and after completing his service he received his Bachelor of Science degree in 1957.

He then went on to earn his Doctor of Medicine Degree from the University of Pittsburgh in 1961. He finished several orthopedic surgical residencies in different parts of the U.S. before setting up practice in Southern California.

He completed an orthopedic surgery residency at Evanston Hospital, Northshore University Health System in Evanston, Illinois as well as one at McGaw Medical Center of Northwestern University in Chicago. He spent a transitional year interning at South Side Hospital in New York.

He was also in the residency program at the Shriners Hospital for Children in Louisville, Kentucky.

Born:	1931
Died:	2021
Years Active:	40+
Location:	Newport Beach, CA
Role(s):	Large Joint Arthroplasty pioneer, associate clinical professor in the Department of Orthopedics, University of California at Irvine

In 1969, Dr. Maravich Newport Beach, California and spent more than 20 years practicing general orthopedic surgery. His California state medical license was active all the way up until his death at age 90.

Anthony F. Merlino

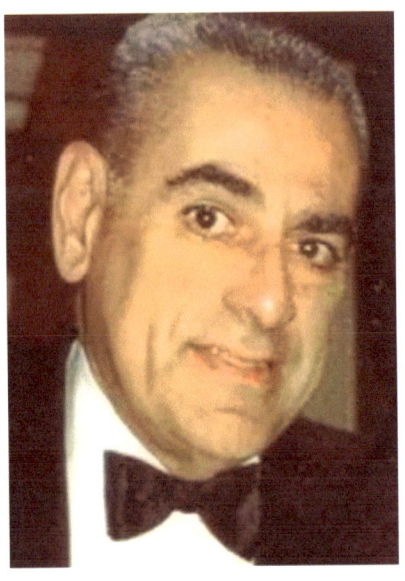

Born:	1930
Died:	2022
Years Active:	40+
Location:	Rhode Island
Role(s):	Co-Founder of the Rhode Island Orthopedic Group, Winner of Providence College's McDonnell Award in 1981 and the Golden Friar Alumni Service Award in 2001 and joint arthroplasty pioneer.

Anthony F. Merlino, M.D., along with his late partners William Hindle, M.D. and Ralph Pike, M.D. founded the Rhode Island Orthopedic Group in North Providence, Rhode Island.

Dr. Merlino was one of the first joint arthroplasty surgeons in Rhode Island and served the greater North Providence area for 40 years practicing at the Fatima and Providence units of St. Joseph Hospital.

Merlino wrote more than 20 scientific articles throughout his extraordinary career. He was also a member of the American Medical Association, American College of Surgeons, American Academy of Orthopedic Surgeons, Rhode Island Orthopedic Society, Eastern Orthopedic Association, Boston Orthopedic Club, and other professional organizations.

He also had a passion for the law and won a few medically oriented cases in both the Rhode Island Supreme Court and the U.S. Supreme Court.

Dr. Merlino spent 20 years as an orthopedic consultant for his alma mater, Providence College, and as a team physician to its NCAA Division I athletic teams. For his dedication, the college honored him with the McDonnell Award in 1981 and the Golden Friar Alumni Service Award in 2001.

He was also recognized in multiple editions of WHO'S WHO IN SCIENCE AND ENGINEERING, WHO'S WHO IN MEDICINE AND HEALTHCARE, WHO'S WHO IN THE EAST, WHO'S

WHO IN AMERICA, and WHO'S WHO IN THE WORLD.

Merlino served his country as a medical officer in the United States Air Force, two years on active duty and then a few years in the Active Reserve.

Merlino was born in Providence to the late Anthony F. and C. Mildren Merlino. After graduating from Classical High School, he went to Providence College, University of Connecticut, and Jefferson Medical College where he pursued a career in orthopedic surgery.

Gary Wayne Miller Sr

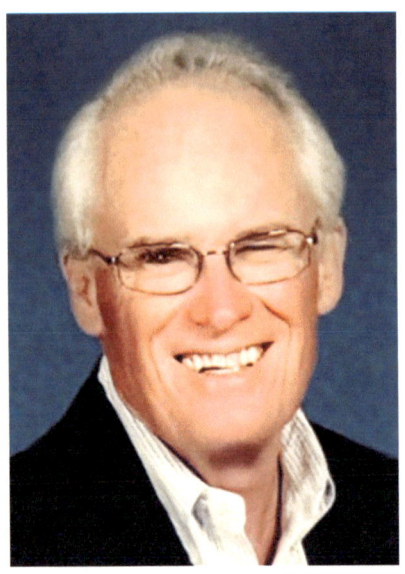

Born:	1944
Died:	2022
Years Active:	45
Location:	Mid-Ohio Valley
Role(s):	Pioneering orthopedic surgeon in the Mid-Ohio Valley

Gary Wayne Miller, Sr., M.D., was one of the first large joint arthroplasty surgeons to set up practice in the mid-Ohio Valley – a geographic region which encompasses a largely rural area of southern Ohio along the Ohio River / West Virginia border.

Dr. Miller was born on June 2, 1944, in Frostburg, Maryland, the son of the late George Charles Miller and Betty Irene Lewis Miller Edwards. After attending high school in Frostburg, he earned his bachelor's degree at West Virginia University and then graduated from the University of Maryland Medical School with his Doctor of Medicine degree.

Miller then went back to West Virginia University for his residency and orthopedic fellowship. He served two years as a doctor in the U.S. Army at Fort Stewart Georgia before setting up his orthopedics practice in the Mid-Ohio Valley.

Miller dedicated 45 years of his life to serving the Mid-Ohio Valley as an orthopedic surgeon.

James E. Mraz

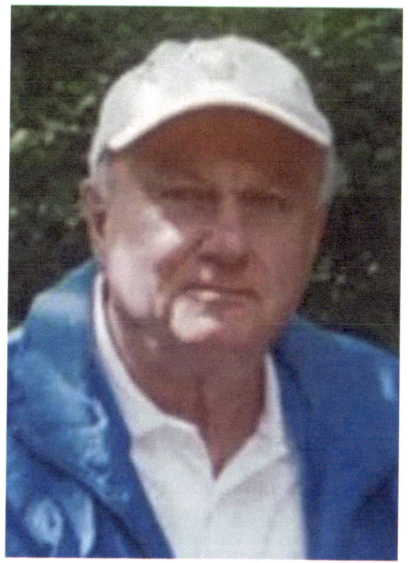

Born:	1936
Died:	2022
Years Active:	30+
Location:	Erie, PA
Role(s):	Pioneering orthopedic surgeon, founding member of Erie, Pa's Orthopedic Surgeons, Inc.

James E. Mraz, M.D., one of the founders of Erie, Pennsylvania's Orthopedic Surgeons, Inc., served the northwest, lakes region Pennsylvania for more than 30 years, was one of the original joint arthroplasty surgeons in the area. Dr. Mraz was affiliated with St. Vincent Hospital and specialized in general orthopedic surgery.

Mraz was born on October 9, 1936, in Erie to the late Dr. John J. and Janette Mraz. He graduated from Cathedral Preparatory School in Erie and then attended Allegheny College in Meadville, Pennsylvania. He earned his medical degree from the University of Pittsburgh Medical School in Pittsburgh.

Dr. Mraz served in the United States Navy for two years after completing his medical degree. He did his orthopedic residency at the University of Buffalo in Buffalo, New York.

Marvin E. Mumme Jr

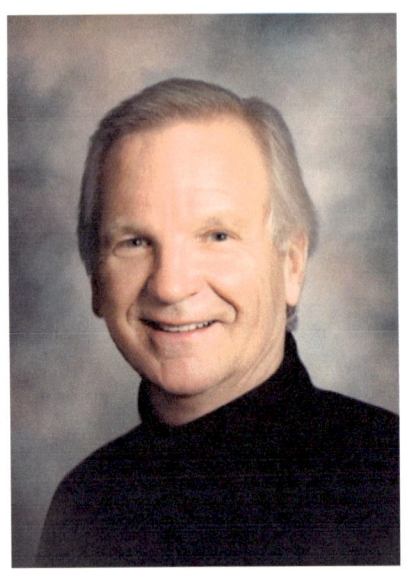

Marvin E. Mumme, Jr., was one of the original large joint arthroplasty surgeons in central Arkansas and spent 38 years with Holt Krock Clinic in Fort Smith, Arkansas, also, about 80 miles away, at Russellville's River Valley Orthopedics and was appointed chief of staff at Sparks Regional Medical Center, also in Fort Smith, and served on the board of trustees as well.

By all accounts, Dr. Mumme was well-loved by his patients and staff and colleagues. In his spare time, he volunteered to be the team doctor for Southside High School football. Before retirement, he also served patients at Mercy Orthopedics, which is part of the River Valley system.

Dr. Mumme was very active in continuing education throughout his career and participated as a diplomate of the American Board of Orthopedic Surgery and a fellow of the American Academy of Orthopedic Surgeons.

Mumme was born in Little Rock, Arkansas, on August 3, 1945, to Lt. Col Marvin Mumme, Sr. and Merle Booe Mumme. He graduated from North Little Rock High School, earned a bachelor's degree from the University of Texas (UT) at Austin and his medical degree from UT Southwestern.

Born:	1945
Died:	2022
Years Active:	38+
Location:	Central Arkansas
Role(s):	Pioneer large joint surgeon, Chief of Staff at Sparks Regional Medical Center and Member of the Board of Trustees.

After completing his residency, he served at Peterson Field Air Force Base in Colorado Springs, Colorado. He was awarded the Medal of Commendation for his service as Assistant Chief of Clinic Services and the excellence of care he provided his patients.

Following his service at Peterson Field, Dr. Mumme settled in Fort Smith, Arkansas as large joint arthroplasty was just working its way from England to the United States.

He was one of the pioneering large joint arthroplasty surgeons in the United States.

Stephen Minick Neely

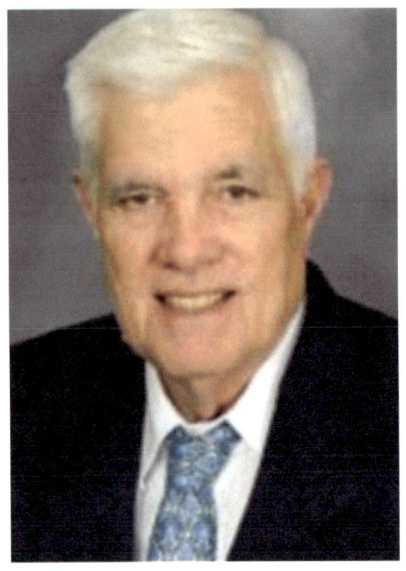

Born:	1945
Died:	2022
Years Active:	20+
Location:	Nashville, TN
Role(s):	Pioneer joint arthroplasty surgeon who performed over 100,000 total joint surgeries.

Orthopedic surgeon Stephen Minick Neely, M.D., was a pioneering joint arthroplasty surgeon, one of the first in Nashville, Tennesee who would over the course of his 20+ year career, perform 10,000 total joint surgeries.

Dr. Neely practiced in the Vanderbilt Wilson County Hospital and the TriStar Summit Medical Center.

Dr. Neely was born on June 1, 1945, in Washington, D.C. to the late Guy Morton and Elizabeth Seymour Neely. He received his medical degree from the University of Virginia School of Medicine and completed his surgical residency at the University of Virginia Medical Center between 1973 and 1975.

Dr. Neely was the first orthopedic surgeon in the Wilson County region, when he moved to Lebanon, Tennessee in 1980.

In addition to his medical practice, Neely was an extraordinarily accomplished mineral collector. His mineral collection can be found in museums around the world.

When he wasn't serving patients, he spent his free time tracking down miners and minerals from the famous Elmwood and Cumberland mines of Tennessee. Sometimes he would exchange his medical services for specimens to add to his collection. Eventually he expanded his mineral collection to include minerals from around the world.

Cecil H. Neville Jr

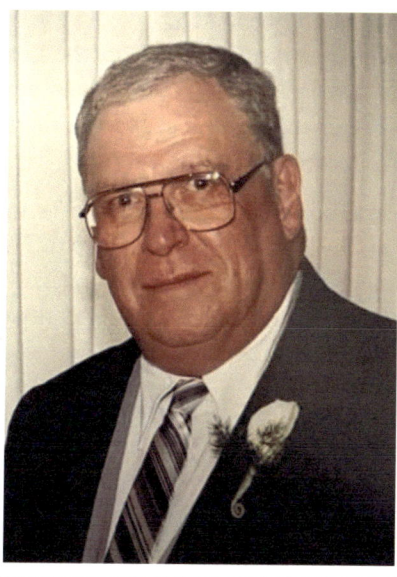

Born:	1935
Died:	2022
Years Active:	30+
Location:	Pinehurst, NC
Role(s):	Founder Pinehurst Orthopedics, Past President North Carolina Orthopedic Association and pioneering orthopedic surgeon.

Cecil H. Neville, Jr., M.D., past president of the North Carolina Orthopedic Association and founder of Pinehurst Orthopedics, was one of the first joint arthroplasty surgeons in North Carolina.

He spent his career in Pinehurst, North Carolina and also started Diagnostic Orthopedics in Fayetteville, North Carolina where he reviewed medical records and served as an expert witness.

Dr. Neville was also past president of the North Carolina Orthopedic Association and as a board member of The O'Neal School in Pinehurst, North Carolina. He served as U.S. Navy physician in both Pensacola, Florida and Norfolk, Virginia.

Neville was born on March 17, 1935, in Scotland Neck, North Carolina to Dr. Cecil Howell Neville, Sr. and Martha Evans Neville.

He grew up in Scotland Neck, attending the high school there. He then graduated from The University of North Carolina at Chapel Hill where he received a Bachelor of Science in Medicine in 1957. Neville earned his medical degree from The University of North Carolina School of Medicine in 1960.

He completed internships and residencies in general and orthopedic surgery at the University of Arkansas and Medical College of Virginia.

Stanford M. Noel

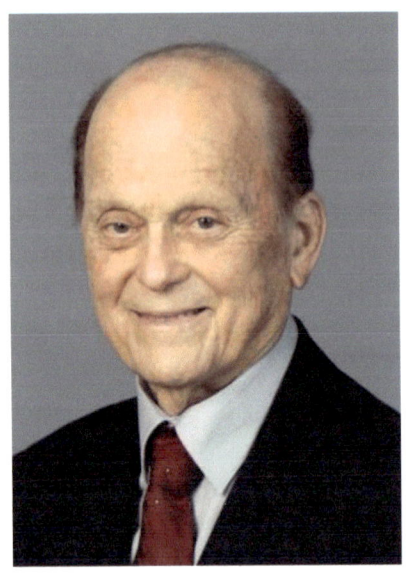

Born:	1935
Died:	2022
Years Active:	50+
Location:	Los Angeles, CA
Role(s):	Pioneer orthopedic surgeon who studied under Dr. John Charnley, President of the Orthopedic Hospital medical staff, orthopedic lobbyist in Congress on behalf of the National Academy of Orthopedic Surgeons

Stanford M. Noel, M.D., was a well-known orthopedic surgeon in the Los Angeles area practicing there for more than 50 years specializing in hip disorders in both children and adults.

Noel was born on December 16, 1934, in Sherman, Texas, to Jewell H. and Oscar H. Noel. He graduated from Rice University with his undergraduate degree and then earned his medical degree at the University of Texas, Galveston.

He then served as a captain in the U.S. Army Medical Corps in Korea as a general surgeon. He spent two years practicing general surgery in Stockton, California, before realizing that his true calling was orthopedics.

He spent one year in research at Harbor General Hospital in Los Angeles, California, and then completed a three-year orthopedic residency at Orthopedic Hospital, also in Los Angeles. He also did a three-year fellowship in hip disorders there as well.

Afterwards, he formed a partnership with Dr. William Craig to treat private patients with hip disorders and together they ran a hip clinic at Orthopedic Hospital for underprivileged children. When Dr. Craig retired, Noel continued the hip clinic and private practice.

He was instrumental in treating challenging and complex hip disorders. Noel was one of the first orthopedic surgeons to study with Dr. John Charnley—arguably the father of hip replacement—in Whittington, England. Noel would later design his own total hip prosthesis for special patient situations.

He was president of the medical staff at Orthopedic Hospital for three terms and was involved in the hospital's teaching program for residents. He was also a member of the National Hip Society. He was chosen as one of two in the state of California for a three-year term as a lobbyist of Congress in Washington representing the National Academy of Orthopedic Surgeons.

Donald Paarlberg

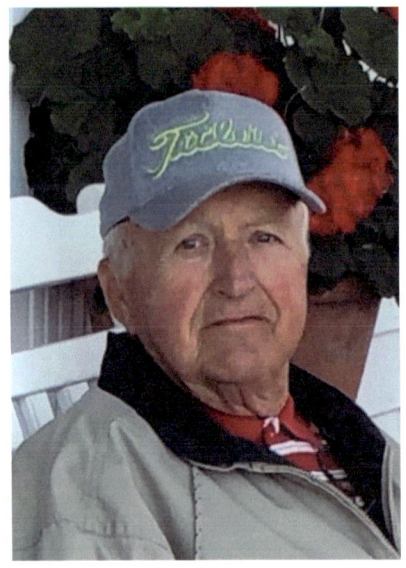

Born:	1937
Died:	2022
Years Active:	30+
Location:	Coldwater, MI
Role(s):	Pioneering joint arthroplasty surgeon and community medical examiner

Donald Paarlberg, M.D., was one of the first large joint arthroplasty surgeons in Greenfield, Massachusetts and, later, Coldwater, Michigan.

He served the southern Michigan area of Coldwater for more than 20 years. He was also his town's medical examiner.

Paarlberg was born on March 21, 1937, in Harvey, Illinois, to Cornelius W. and Herminia Shilling Paarlberg. He graduated from Hope College and then earned his medical degree at Northwestern Medical School. To further his training, he did an orthopedic surgery residency at the Mayo Clinic Minnesota.

During the Vietnam War, Paarlberg was drafted into the U.S. Army, the 82nd Airborne, as medical doctor and served from 1964-1966. Afterwards, he set up a private practice in Greenfield, Massachusetts, and then relocated to Coldwater. He ran his Coldwater practice from 1978 to 2000.

Mark Palumbo

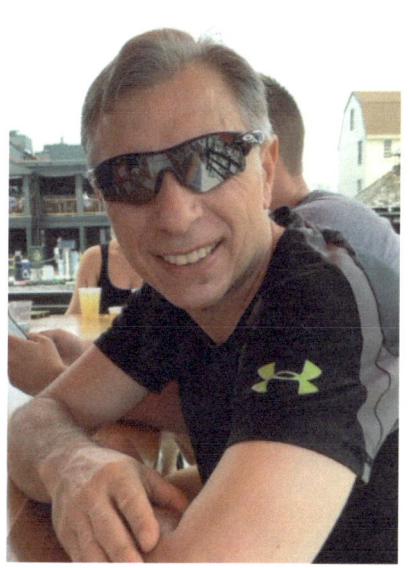

Born:	1962
Died:	2019
Years Active:	25+
Location:	Rhode Island
Role(s):	Chief Emeritus, Division of Spine Surgery Professor of Orthopedic Surgery, Brown University, Director, Brown University Fellowship in Spine Surgery Vice President, University Orthopedics Incorporated

Dr. Mark A. Palumbo was a practicing Spine Surgeon for over 25 years, Chief of Spine Surgery at Rhode Island Hospital and recipient of many Academic Honor Awards during his medical career – notably the Award for Excellence in Teaching-Brown University Orthopedic Residency Program.

Dr. Palumbo was recently honored for several AAOS Achievement Awards 2018-19. He published and co-published over 70 publications for medical journals. Dr. Palumbo was a true mentor, healer, teacher and loyal friend to so many.

Mark was born on January 29th, 1962, in Providence, RI to Ralph and Marie (Mallette) Palumbo.

Mark graduated from Bishop Hendricken High School ('80'), Boston University, Magna Cum Laude ('84'), Boston University Medical School ('88). Soon after, Mark became a resident at Rhode Island Hospital/Brown University Medical Program. His specialty was Spine Surgery where he attended the Case Western Reserve University Spine Fellowship Program.

University Orthopedics Inc. (UOI), based in East Providence, Rhode Island, where Dr. Palumbo treated many of his patients, renamed its annual fund-raising 5K run after Dr. Palumbo.

Funds raised from the Mark Palumbo Memorial University Orthopedics 5K went to The Tomorrow Fund, a non-profit organization that provides financial and emotional support for children being treated for cancer at Hasbro Children's Hospital and their families.

"Dr. Palumbo improved the lives of countless patients throughout his esteemed career. He was not only an accomplished surgeon but a true leader and someone who inspired many in the field of medicine," said University Orthopedics President Dr. Edward Akelman.

Victor Panitch

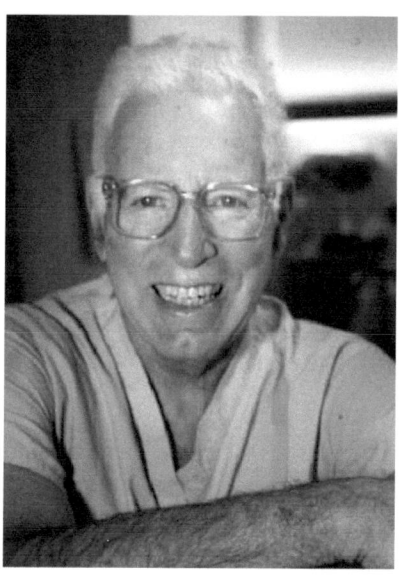

Born:	1932
Died:	2022
Years Active:	40+
Location:	Holyoke, MA
Role(s):	Pioneering orthopedic surgeon, President of the orthopedic staff at both Holyoke and Providence Hospitals, founder of the scoliosis screening program for Holyoke public schools.

Victor Panitch, M.D., a long-time orthopedic physician at Shriner's Hospital for Children in Holyoke, Massachusetts, was also president of the staff at both Holyoke and Providence Hospitals and as a member of the board of directors at both hospitals.

Panitch was a well-loved and respected orthopedic surgeon in the Holyoke community of central Massachusetts. He served all of Hampden country and, notably, Springfield, Massachusetts through his private practice, Holyoke Orthopedics Inc., and as a staff member of the Holyoke and Providence Hospitals. He was also, by invitation, an attending staff member at Shriners Hospital for Children.

Dr. Panitch volunteered at Shriner's Hospital and traveled to other countries and across New England to identify children with unmet orthopedic needs and to provide care for them, or to help facilitate treatment at the specialist hospital in Springfield, Massachusetts. He volunteered with Shriner's until he retired.

Dr. Panitch also founded the scoliosis screening program for the Holyoke public schools and served on the board of directors of the Newell C. Mansir Trust.

For his commitment to helping others, Panitch was the inaugural recipient of the Holyoke Medical Center and Holyoke Hospital Auxiliary Distinguished Service Award in 2014.

Panitch who was born in 1932 grew up in Irvington, New Jersey, and graduated from Irvington High School in 1950. He then graduated from Franklin and Marshall College in Lancaster, Pennsylvania, in 1954 and then attended Jefferson Medical College in Philadelphia. He earned his medical degree in 1958.

While in school, he was inducted into Alpha Omega Alpha, the National Medical Honor Society. He did his orthopedic residency with the Lahey Clinic in Burlington, Massachusetts, from 1962 to 1965.

Panitch served his country in the U.S. Navy at Mystic, Connecticut, submarine base. Additionally, he served with U.S. Marines at Camp Lejeune, North Carolina.

Dr. Panitch was a man of eclectic interests and wide-ranging expertise. He could fly an airplane, tie a fly, keep bees, bake sourdough bread, and, if necessary, perform surgery on a child's pet goose.

John P. Park

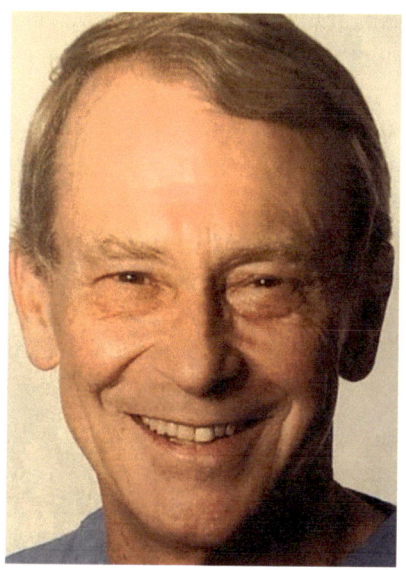

Born:	1947
Died:	2022
Years Active:	
Location:	Northwest Arkansas
Role(s):	Pioneering orthopedic surgeon, team physician Arkansas Razorback football team and Arkansas representative to the American Association of Sports Medicine Association

John P. Park, M.D., was the team physician for the Arkansas Razorback football team for more than 30 years. In his day job, he was a pioneering large joint and sports medicine physician in northwest Arkansas.

Dr. Park was born May 15, 1947, in La Junta, Colorado. He attended college and medical school at the University of Washington and graduated in 1972.

Dr. Park completed his surgical residency at Strong Memorial Hospital in Rochester, New York, and his orthopedic surgical residency at UAMS in Little Rock, Arkansas. He then participated in a sports medicine fellowship at Slocum and Larsen Clinic in Oregon.

Dr. Park was a member of Ozark Orthopedics in Fayetteville and was affiliated with Northwest Medical Center-Springdale and Washington Regional Medical Center. He also was the voluntary team physician for the Arkansas Razorbacks for more than 30 years.

After retiring, Park spent five years as the medical director at Tyson Foods. He also spent time as the Arkansas representative for the American Orthopedic Society for Sports Medicine and served on the Governor's Council for Physical Fitness in Arkansas.

Preston Philips

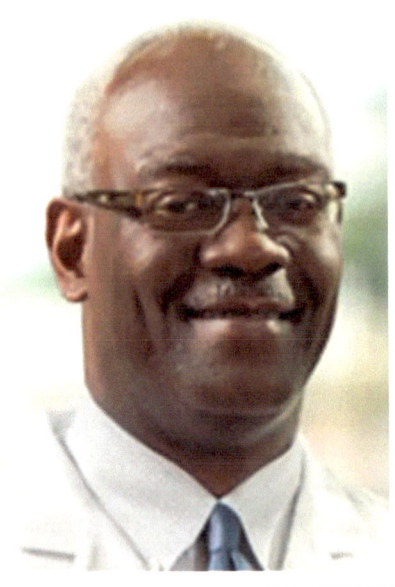

Born:	1963
Died:	2022
Years Active:	25
Location:	Tulsa, OK
Role(s):	Spine surgeon at St. Francis Hospital, Tulsa Oklahoma, emeritus board member of Saint Francis Health System in Tulsa, Board member John Hope Franklin Center for Reconciliation, Team physician for the Women's National Basketball Association's Tulsa Shock

Preston Phillips MD, a Harvard Medical School (HMS) graduate with honors, was a Tulsa, Oklahoma based spine surgeon who was a notably consequential leader in the broader orthopedic and spine community.

After graduating from HMS, Dr. Phillips completed an orthopedic residency at Yale as well as fellowships at Beth Israel Deaconess Medical Center and Boston Children's Hospital.

While at Harvard, he worked with Augustus White III, the Ellen and Melvin Gordon Distinguished Professor of Medical Education and an HMS professor of orthopedic surgery at Beth Israel Deaconess; together they produced a book on back pain written for the lay public.

Phillips also earned advanced degrees in organic chemistry and pharmacology and theology from Emory University.

In addition to being a skilled orthopedic surgeon who specialized in spine disorders, joint reconstruction, and surgical procedures, Phillips was a fellow of the American Orthopedic Association, the Scoliosis Research Society, the American Academy of Orthopaedic Surgeons, and the J. Robert Gladden Orthopaedic Society, which works to increase diversity in orthopedics.

He was a member of the board of directors of the John Hope Franklin Center for Reconciliation, which works to transform social divisions into social harmony in memory of those lost in the 1921 race massacre in Tulsa.

At the Franklin Center, he chaired its scholarship committee, recruiting fellow members of his fraternity for Black professionals, called Grand Boule of the Sigma Pi Phi Fraternity (Epsilon Iota), to review applications, nominate students for awards and mentor the winners through post-secondary education

He was also the former team physician for the Tulsa Shock, part of the Women's National Basketball Association.

In addition, Phillips participated in medical missions to Togo, Africa, organized by the Tulsa-based Light in the World Development Foundation. Along with fellow Saint Francis physician, Komi Folley, M.D., an internist, he helped build clinics and hospitals, practice medicine and bring supplies.

In fact, Dr. Phillips donated several containers of prosthetics for knee replacement for the surgical team.

Preston Phillips was born in 1963 into a family that would eventually be 9 children. He grew up in both Saginaw, Michigan and Atlanta, Georgia.

His brother, Phil, who is a partner in the Detroit law firm of Foley & Lardner LLP, recalls entering Emory University after his older brother Preston. "In four years at Emory Preston graduated with a bachelor's degree in theology, a bachelor's degree in chemistry and a master's in organic chemistry. So, when I got to Emory and they said, 'You're Preston Phillips' brother.' I said, 'I'm here for one degree. I am not Preston.' I think he studied more in high school than I probably did in law school. I mean, he was just off the charts."

After Emory, Dr. Phillips was accepted to Harvard Medical School and graduated with honors in 1992.

From 1998 to 2005, he was on staff at Swedish Medical Center with Seattle Orthopedics.

Dr. Phillips was a mountain of a man who gave up playing basketball to focus on his studies at Harvard.

In June 2022 a spine patient named Michael Louis, who was 2 weeks into his surgical recovery, but blamed Dr. Phillips for the pain he was still experiencing, went to Dr. Phillip's south Tulsa clinic and shot Dr. Phillips, a second doctor, a receptionist and another patient to death before killing himself before police arrived. It was the 233rd mass shooting of 2022.

Thomas Lemuel Presson

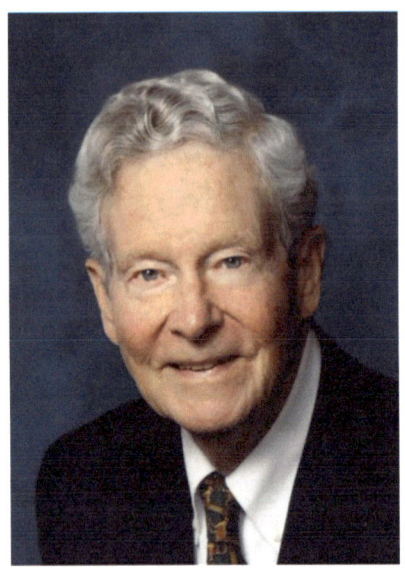

Born:	1940
Died:	2022
Years Active:	30+
Location:	Greensboro, NC
Role(s):	President, North Carolina Orthopaedic Association, Pioneer orthopedic surgeon, UNC Morehead Scholar

Thomas Lemuel Presson, M.D. was a member of and practiced at the Greensboro Orthopedic Clinic for more than 30 years serving patients throughout the triad region of Greensboro, Winston-Salem, and High Point, North Carolina.

Dr. Presson earned his medical degree at the University of North Carolina at Chapel Hill where he was selected to be a Morehead Scholar—the first national merit scholarship program established at a public university.

The Morehead scholar's program was designed to recognize young student leaders who have the demonstrated ability to influence, energize, and inspire others to make an impact. The selection committee choose young students who have demonstrated courage, humility, integrity, and perseverance as well as an authentic love of learning and of sharing that newfound knowledge and inspiration with others.

Throughout his 30+ year career, Dr. Presson demonstrated amply the qualities that, at an early age, had impressed the Morehead Scholar selection committee.

Dr. Presson was also an active member of the Southern Orthopaedic Association, the Atlantic Bone Club, and the North Carolina Orthopaedic Association. He served a term as president for the North Carolina Orthopaedic Association.

Presson was born on May 6, 1940, in Monroe, North Carolina, to Rosa Nell Cox Presson and Lawrence Stewart Presson. He graduated from Walter Bickett High School in Monroe and then earned his bachelor's degree at the University of North Carolina at Chapel Hill, where he also attended medical school.

After medical school, he served as a major at the United States Army and was based in Frankfurt, Germany, between 1967 and 1970.

Gurdev Purewal

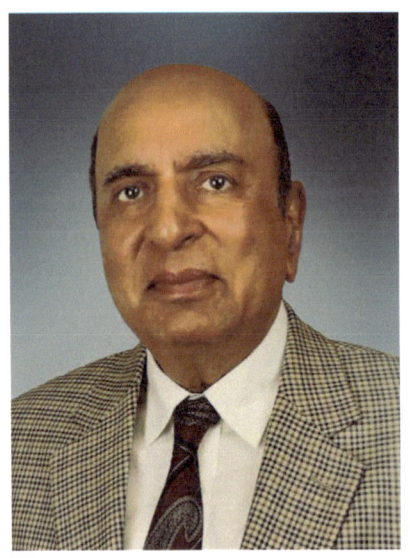

Born:	1938
Died:	2020
Years Active:	40+
Location:	Weirton, WV
Role(s):	President of the Weirton Medical Center and member of the Medical Center's Board of Trustees. Pioneer orthopedic surgeon.

Gurdev Purewal MD, was a pioneer orthopedic surgeon and served the broader community of Weirton, West Virginia and Steubenville, Ohio for , more than 40 years.

Born in Kalewal in Hoshiarpur, a small village in northern India, he was the youngest of five children.

Purewal attended a local school until the fifth grade, then was accepted to the Lawrence School Sanawar before doing his pre-med studies at the University of Allahabad. He spent a year at St. Xavier's College in Ranchi before going to medical school at Government College Medical School at Amritsar, India.

He worked for several years as a lecturer in orthopedic surgery and trained for three years at the Royal Orthopedic Hospital in Birmingham, England, before returning to India and being promoted to assistant professor at his medical school and then moving to the United States in 1975, along with his wife, Surinderit, and their three children.

Purewal did a two-year residency at Hamot Medical Center in Erie, Pa., then moved to Weirton, West Virginia, a community about 40 miles due west of Pittsburgh, Pennsylvania in 1977.

Dr. Purewal joined the Weirton Medical Center staff in 1977. He would eventually become president of the Weirton Medical Center and a member of its board of trustees.

He was not only a physician and one of the first orthopedic surgeons in the area, but Dr. Purewal was also a civic leader, said John Frankovitch, president and CEO of Weirton Medical Center.

"Dr. Purewal was a complete professional in every aspect of his medical practice as well as in his personal life, serving as a role model to others. His gentle, friendly demeanor matched with exceptional medical ability was truly a gift to WMC and our patients for over 40 years. Purewal had the unique ability to make us smile in difficult times but challenge us to find our 'better angels' in our daily lives."

Purewal was active in the Weirton community, as well, lending his time to organizations such as the Weirton Rotary Club, where he was past president. It was through that work for the community, Purewal was inducted as a member of the Weirton Hall of Fame in 2018.

During his 2018 induction into the Weirton Hall of Fame, Purewal explained he often told his staff not to bill patients who couldn't afford medical services saying he "didn't want to make money off people who couldn't make a living."

Mario Randelli

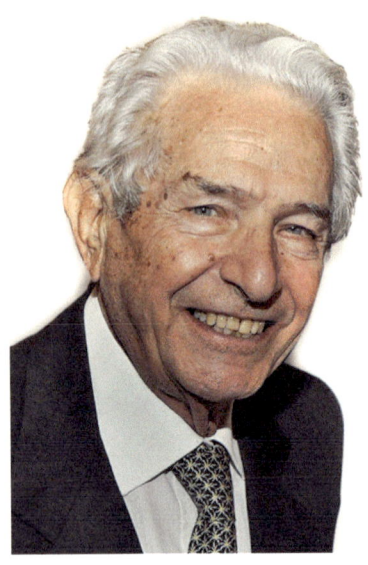

Born:	1928
Died:	2020
Years Active:	40+
Location:	Villanova, Italy
Role(s):	Inventor of the "Randelli" anatomical system, president of the Italian Society of Orthopedics and Traumatology, founder and president of the Italian Shoulder and Elbow Society and the European Society of Surgery of the Shoulder and the Elbow

Professor Mario Randelli is perhaps best known for his work with LimaCorporate, the northern Italian orthopedic product manufacturer. He is also, among his very many accomplishments, the developer of the "Randelli" anatomical system.

Professor Randelli was also instrumental in the development of LimaCorporate's SMR Modular Shoulder System in 2002. A member of the Clinical Institute Humanitas of Milan at the time, he led a group of shoulder surgeons in support of its development.

"I would like to remember him with his sentence – '[...] it is important to have access not only to a single modular solution but to a system which will allow the switch from an implant to the other even during surgery' – This revolutionary statement led to the development of a revolutionary system that today allows a greater intraoperative versatility and a better result for the patient, who can thus be treated in a very specific way," said Luigi Ferrari, chief executive officer of LimaCorporate.

Professor Randelli performed over 20,000 orthopedic and trauma surgeries. He was also the author of over 90 publications.

A strong leader in many ways, he was the president of the Italian Society of Orthopedics and Traumatology, founder and president of the Italian Shoulder and Elbow Society and the European Society of Surgery of the Shoulder and the Elbow.

"I am very proud to say Prof. Randelli has been at our side in the development of one our most successful systems. His pioneering vision and his approach to innovation will continue to be a source of inspiration for all of us," said Ferrari.

John F. Raycroft

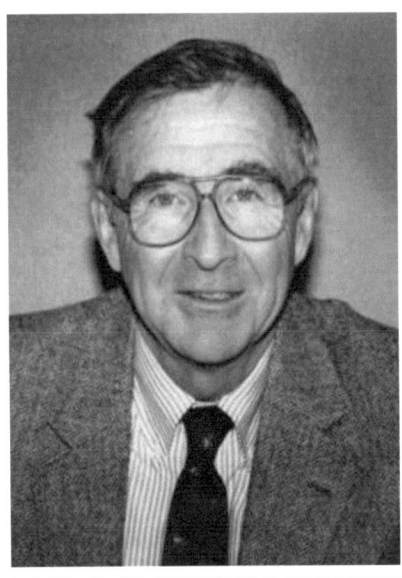

Born:	1931
Died:	2022
Years Active:	59+
Location:	Hartford, CT
Role(s):	Founder of the Orthopedic Associates of Hartford, Professor of orthopedics at University of Connecticut and Yale University

John F. Raycroft, M.D., was a pioneering orthopedic surgeon in Connecticut and founded the Orthopedic Associates of Hartford. For more than 50 years. Dr. Raycroft treated patients at the Hartford Hospital, Newington Children's Hospital and was a member of the medical school faculty at both the University of Connecticut and Yale University.

Dr. Raycroft was also a member of the executive leadership for both the New England Orthopedic Society and the Yale Orthopedic Association.

Dr. Raycroft also ran the local Grange annual fair in the early 1970s and in 1993, he organized a parade for the town's tricentennial celebration. He was also a member of Glastonbury's Historical Society and helped organized house and garden tours and the society's fundraising efforts.

For many summers, Dr. Raycroft would take his doctor bag up to Camp Dudley in Westport, NY, serving as camp doctor for a period.

Raycroft was born on April 27, 1931, in Brooklyn, New York, to the late John F. and Ruth Raycroft. His father was chief of surgery at Kings County Hospital in Brooklyn and greatly influenced his life's work.

After graduating from Poly Prep Day School, he went to Syracuse University for geography. He then served in the U.S. Navy for four years.

It was then he enrolled in medical school at SUNY Downstate and received his medical degree in 1961. He then completed an orthopedic surgery internship and residency at Yale New Haven Hospital between 1961 and 1963.

Next he spent three years at Newington Children's Hospital furthering his training.

Robert Ernest Ribbe

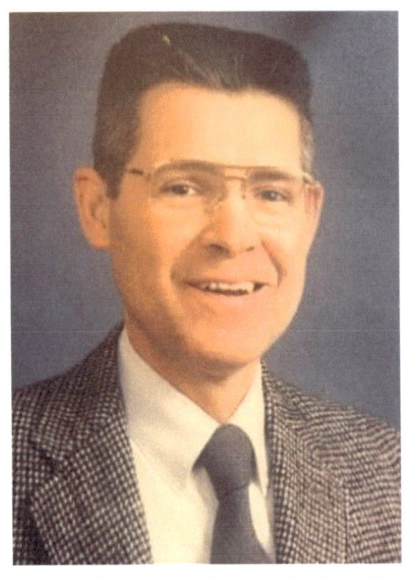

Born:	1937
Died:	2022
Years Active:	26+
Location:	Grand Rapids, MI
Role(s):	Pioneer orthopedic surgeon, volunteer surgeon in Kenya, Romania, Taiwan and for 20 years inmates of the Michigan prison system and a Vietnam Vet

Robert Ernest Ribbe, M.D., a Vietnam Vet and orthopedic surgeon, treated patients for more than thirty years in and around Grand Rapids, Michigan but also, as a volunteer surgeon, in Kenya, Romania, Taiwan and, for 20 years, patients in Michigan's prison system.

Ribbe was born in 1937 in Patterson, New Jersey, to Reverend Walter and Grace Ribbe. He graduated from Wheaton College with a bachelor's degree in chemistry. While there, he was a member of the Army ROTC.

After Wheaton, Ribbe attended University of Pennsylvania Medical School and graduated with his medical degree.

Dr. Ribbe's residency in general surgery was at Ft. Knox, Kentucky, where he was serving in the U.S. Army. He also entered the residency in orthopedic surgery program at Tripler Army Hospital, then a residency at Shriner's Children Hospital in Honolulu, Hawaii, and an internship at Madigan Army Hospital in Tacoma, Washington.

Ribbe served in the Vietnam war from 1968 to 1969. He was deployed to the 311th Field Hospital.

After Vietnam, Dr. Ribbe was stationed at the West Point Army Hospital. In 1971, he moved his family to Grand Rapids, Michigan, where he was a senior staff member in the orthopedic surgery department at the Butterworth Hospital, where he stayed until he retired in 1994.

Ribbe was a member of the Christian Medical/Dental Society through which he volunteered his medical skills to treat patients at no charge in Kenya, Romania, and

Taiwan. He also spent almost 20 years ministering to prisoners. He and his wife extended their personal ministry to international students from Grand Valley State University.

Sheldon Roger

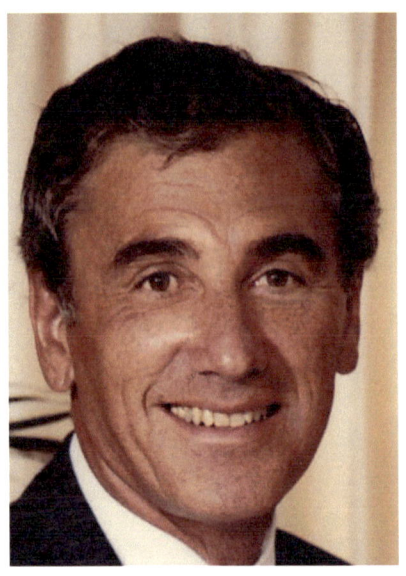

Born:	1930
Died:	2016
Years Active:	50+
Location:	Denver, CO
Role(s):	Orthopedic physician for the Denver Nugget professional basketball team, Chief of Orthopedics at the VA System in Colorado, pioneer orthopedic surgeon in Denver.

Sheldon Roger, M.D., was best known as the team physician for the Denver Nuggets NBA team. He was also the Chief of Orthopedics at the massive Veterans Affairs hospital in the Denver area and served that community for nearly half a century.

Dr. Roger earned his medical degree at Indiana University and then completed his surgical residency at Mount Sinai Hospital in New York City.

He served as a captain in the U.S. Army medical corps from 1955 to 1957. After that, with joint arthroplasty just emerging from Britain, Dr. Roger entered the young orthopedic residency program in 1960 at the University of Colorado School of Medicine.

He practiced orthopedics at Rose Medical Center and at the Veterans Administration Hospital. In 1997 and 1998, he was asked to be the VA's chief of orthopedics.

Dr. Roger's son, Stephen, said of his father, "He had a private practice for over 50 years. I truly enjoyed spending hours in his office and watching him work. Medicine was really a 'calling' for my dad. At times, my dad would stop by a patient's house every day to see how they were doing."

"Sports medicine gave him a real thrill, and he knew that he was fortunate to be able to bring these two worlds together. I think one of his favorite periods as a physician was when he was with the Denver Nuggets.

Raymond Donald Santucci

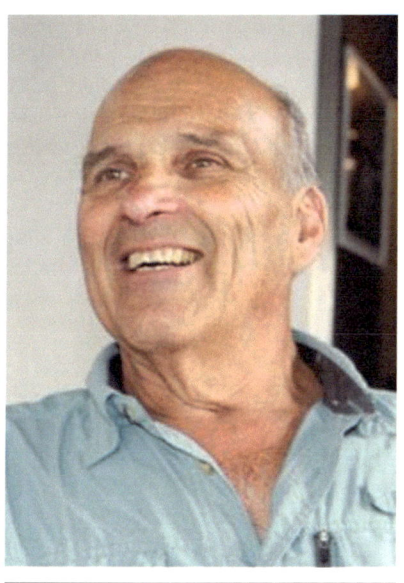

Born:	1942
Died:	2022
Years Active:	40+
Location:	Winfield-Wheaton, IL
Role(s):	Assistant Professor of orthopedic surgery at Loyola University Hospital and Shriners Crippled Children's Hospital in Oak Park, Illinois, Chief of Orthopedics and President of the Medical Staff Central DuPage Hospital.

Raymond Donald Santucci, M.D., graduated from medical school just as joint arthroplasty was being introduced to the United States.

He was one of the early orthopedic surgeons in the Winfield-Wheaton suburbs of Chicago and ultimately dedicated his life to a series and variety of volunteer organizations – two of which he helped found.

Along the way, he plied his orthopedic surgery and other medical skills at mission hospitals around the world, taught future surgeons as assistant professor of orthopedic surgery at Loyola University Hospital and Shriners Crippled Children's Hospital in Oak Park, Illinois and mentored up and coming surgeons as chief of orthopedics and president of the medical staff at Central DuPage Hospital.

Santucci was born to Guido and Ernestine Santucci on April 22, 1941, in Chicago, Illinois. He graduated from Fenwick High School in Oak Park, where he won a Catholic League Football Championship.

He then received his undergraduate degree from Loyola University in 1963 and his medical degree from Loyola Stritch School of Medicine in 1967.

After an internship, he served in the Navy as Lt. Commander and was a combat orthopedic surgeon at the DaNang Naval Hospital in Vietnam.

Once he completed his orthopedic residency, he opened his private practice in the Winfield-Wheaton area of Illinois.

Santucci was a fellow to the American Academy of Orthopaedic Surgery. He retired from private practice in 1999 and then moved to Florida where he served at the VA Hospital in Fort Myers.

His volunteering never stopped. He was instrumental in launching a volunteer organization, the Medical Reserve Corps, in both Southwest Florida and Illinois.

He also became an instructor with the American Medical Association where he educated other physicians, first responders, and healthcare professionals about providing medical care in the event of terrorist attacks or other disasters.

Dr. Santucci's story was a demonstration of living a value-driven life. His mother had died when Dr. Santucci was a young boy. He was raised by aunts and uncles and learned about his Italian ancestry, embracing a life built upon the values of his Catholic faith.

He worked hard to achieve his success. From his teens on through medical school, he toiled to make ends meet, working as a plumber, carpenter, a soda jerk, a Chicago City bus driver, and even setting up pins at the bowling alley.

Francis (Frank) Henry Schildgen

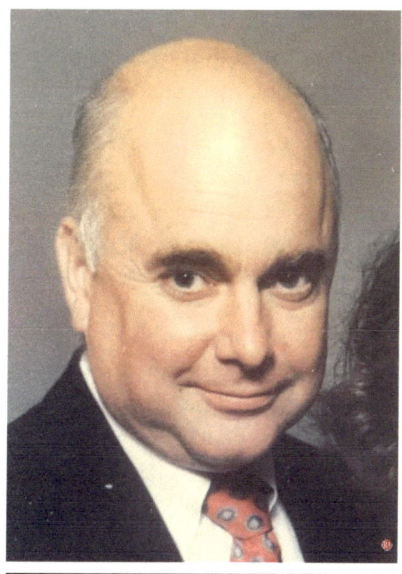

Born:	1947
Died:	2022
Years Active:	37
Location:	Torrington, CT
Role(s):	Pioneer orthopedic surgeon

Francis (Frank) Henry Schildgen, M.D., was one of the first large joint arthroplasty surgeons in the Torrington, Connecticut region and served the area for 37 years.

After retiring, continued to be active in the operations of the Charlotte Hungerford Hospital Orthopedic Clinic. He believed that everyone deserved to get the medical care they needed regardless of the cost, and never turned away a patient who was unable to pay for treatment.

Schildgen was born on November 8, 1946, to the late Francis and Sarah Schildgen. He attended Naugatuck public schools and then received his bachelor's degree from the University of Connecticut.

After graduation, he earned his medical degree at the New Jersey College of Medicine and then went on to complete a residency in orthopedic surgery through Boston University.

R.J. Black Schultz

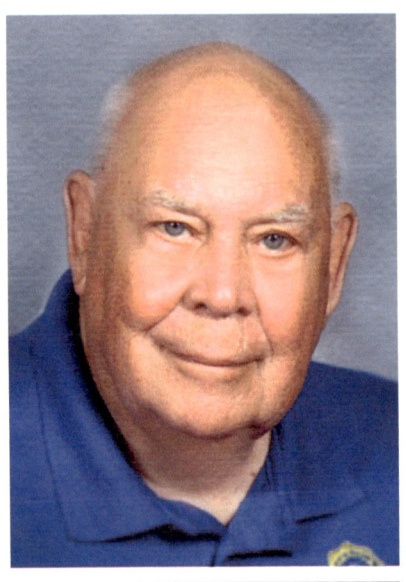

Born:	1933
Died:	2016
Years Active:	30+
Location:	Pueblo and Colorado Springs, CO
Role(s):	Chief of orthopedic surgery at the Air Force Academy

R.J. Black Schultz, M.D. was the chief of orthopedic surgery at the Air Force Academy in Colorado Springs, Colorado.

A native Oklahoman, Dr. Schultz was commander of an Air Force surgical team in the Vietnam delta, service that resulted in his earning both a Bronze Star and the Air Medal.

After leading the department of orthopedic surgery at the Air Force Academy, Dr. Schultz continued his work as one of the first orthopedic surgeons in Pueblo, Colorado where he treated patients for 26 years, 1971 to 1997.

Dr. Schultz was a co-founder of the Pueblo Historical Aviation Society and was active in the Air Force Association, American Legion Post 2, Eagles, VFW and other veterans' groups, Greater Pueblo Chamber of Commerce, Pueblo Economic Development Corporation, Investors Club, and Boy Scouts.

Retired Col. John Feagin, Jr., M.D., former Hospital Commander at West Point said of Dr. Schultz, "He was a legend. He was an outstanding and inspiring Team Physician at the Air Force Academy, and I visited him while I was in the same position at West Point. I was much impressed."

Sidney Schultz

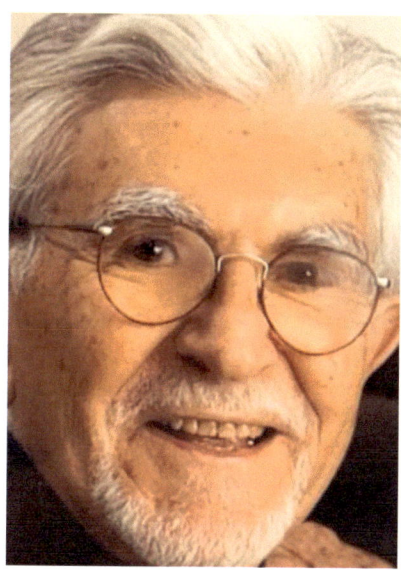

Born:	1921
Died:	2022
Years Active:	
Location:	Albuquerque, NM
Role(s):	Performed First Total Hip Replacement in New Mexico

Sidney Schultz, M.D. of Albuquerque, New Mexico performed the first total hip replacement in New Mexico. It should be also noted, he lived past 100 years of age.

Schulz often called orthopedic surgeons "sterile carpenters." But what made him truly remarkable the people who knew him best say is his compassion and empathy for his patients and among his colleagues, he was renowned for his operating room skills.

One patient wrote him a poem that he kept on his office wall: "A patient's plea: When I am stricken knee, hip and thigh Or wounded grievously do I lie. I pray that God will send to me Schultz's artistic surgery!"

Schulz was also a well-respected expert medical witness who had a knack for putting complicated medical terminology into easily understandable language.

Schulz was born in New Jersey but moved to Albuquerque after finishing his medical residency in Louisiana at Tulane University. A few years later he opened his own practice.

His medical degree is from St. Louis University School of Medicine. He also completed a residency in general surgery at Montefiore Medical Center/Albert Einstein College of Medicine and an internal medicine at New York Downtown Hospital. He did a transitional year internship with Interfaith Medical Center.

Richard E. Senghas

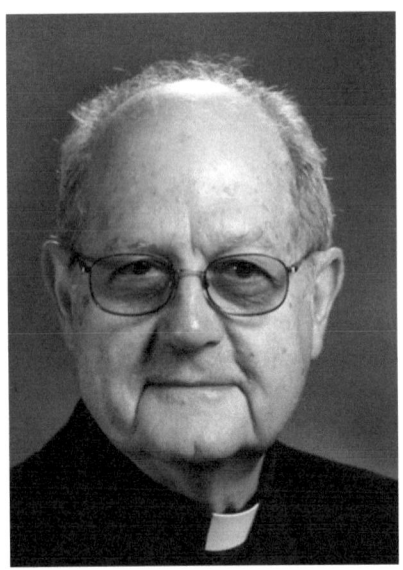

Born:	1928
Died:	2022
Years Active:	
Location:	Middlesex County, MA
Role(s):	President of the medical staff Framingham Union Hospital, Instructor University of Massachusetts Medical School, member of the editorial board Journal of Bone and Joint Surgery and Catholic Priest.

Richard E. Senghas, M.D., was a pioneer orthopedic surgeon in Middlesex county, a western suburb of Boston, Massachusetts, one of the leading orthopedic instructors in the Boston area and, later in life, a Catholic Priest.

Senghas was born on June 30, 1928, in Cleveland, Ohio, to Erwin William Senghas and Lydia Mueller Senghas. He graduated from Lakewood High School in Lakewood, Ohio, and then graduated from Harvard College in Boston, Massachusetts, in 1950 and received his medical degree from Harvard Medical School in 1954.

In January 1955, Senghas married Gertrude (June) June Murray, one of his medical school classmates. They started their internships in Cleveland and then soon departed for Japan where he was a medical officer for the Navy in Yokosuka and June worked as a pediatrician on the Army base in Yokohama.

When they returned to Cleveland, they completed their internships and eventually settled back in the Boston area. Senghas completed his training in orthopedic surgery at Children's Hospital and Massachusetts General Hospital.

In 1963, he joined Framingham Orthopedic Associates, a private orthopedic surgical practice affiliated with Framingham Union Hospital (now MetroWest Medical Center).

Senghas also served as president of the medical staff at Framingham Union Hospital, attending physician at Bethany Hospital, and a clinical instructor at University of Massachusetts Medical School in Worcester.

He was on the editorial board for the *Journal of Bone & Joint Surgery* and volunteered on the Hopkinton Board of Health. He retired from orthopedic surgery in 1988.

After his wife died in 1993, Dr. Senghas entered Pope St. John XXIII National Seminary in Weston, Massachusetts, and served as a chaplain intern for both Wellesley College and Central Maine Medical Center in Lewiston, Maine. At the age of 70, in 1998, he was ordained as a Catholic priest for the Diocese of Maine.

Dr. Senghas's twin brother Robert preceded him as an ordained Catholic priest

He served in St. John the Evangelist and Holy Cross Parishes in South Portland and St. Rose of Lima in Jay. He was also an officer of Ecumenical and Interreligious Affairs for the Catholic diocese of Portland and served on the board of the Maine Council of Churches.

Because of his perspective as a medical doctor and priest, he became an advocate in Augusta, the capital city of Maine, and testified on important legislative issues including climate change and the expansion of Medicaid, emphasizing that healthcare is an important human right.

John "Jack" Haines Shertzer

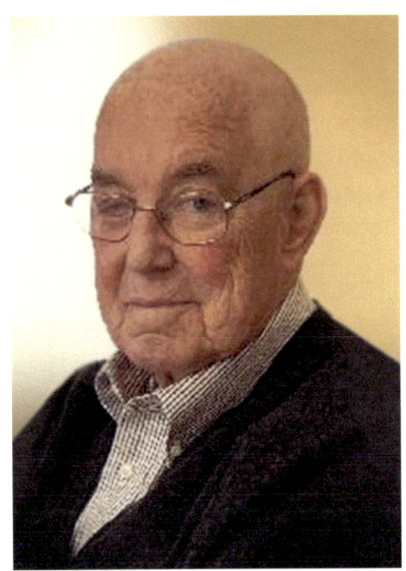

Born:	1938
Died:	2022
Years Active:	40+
Location:	Lancaster, PA
Role(s):	Co-founder of Orthopaedic Associates of Lancaster, Pennsylvania, pioneer orthopedic surgeon and chief of orthopedics and member of the Board of Directors at Lancaster General Hospital.

John "Jack" Haines Shertzer, M.D., orthopedic surgeon, was a pioneering orthopedic surgeon in central Pennsylvania and co-founder of Orthopaedic Associates of Lancaster.

Dr. Shertzer and Dr. Alfred Cooke started Orthopedic Associates of Lancaster, Pennsylvania—in Lancaster, one of the oldest towns in the United States—in 1972 and the practice celebrated its 50th anniversary this year.

Drs. Shertzer and Cooke introduced the practice of joint replacement surgery to central Pennsylvania. Prior to starting Orthopedic Associates with Cooke, Shertzer worked with Dr. William G. Phippen.

Dr. Shertzer also served as chief of orthopedics and chief of staff at Lancaster General Hospital where he was a member of the hospital board of directors from 1986 to 1996. In 2015, Shertzer was inducted into Lancaster General Hospital's Societas Generalis for his commitment and service to the hospital and his patients.

He earned his bachelor's degree from Swarthmore College. Shertzer received his medical degree from Temple Medical School in 1964 and completed his internship at Lancaster General Hospital from 1964 to 1965. He then did his orthopedic residency from 1965 to 1969 at the Mayo Clinic.

After medical school, he served in the U.S. Army at Fort Bragg, North Carolina, for two years where he earned the rank of Major.

Shertzer was born in Lancaster to the late Charles Haines and Kathyrn Shertzer. He attended J.P. McCaskey High School where he served as class president and graduated as the valedictorian of his class in 1956.

Shertzer was also an athlete in school. He was a two-time Pennsylvania Interscholastic Athletic Association, Inc. tennis champion and was named outstanding athlete at McCaskey. He was inducted into the McCaskey Athletic Hall of Fame in 1995 and was honored by the Lancaster County Tennis Hall of Fame in 2016.

William H. Simon

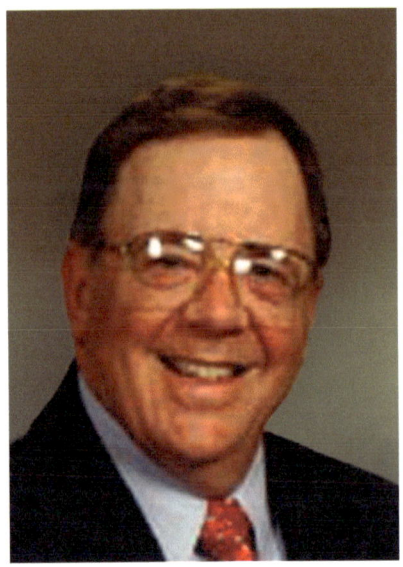

Born:	1938
Died:	2022
Years Active:	40+
Location:	Villanova, PA
Role(s):	Pioneer orthopedic surgeon and author of numerous studies at the National Institutes of Health on the subject of arthritis and metabolic disease.

William H. Simon, M.D was among the earliest large joint arthroplasty surgeons along the Main Line just outside of Philadelphia as well as singer and mystery novel writer.

Dr. Simon spent his entire surgical and teaching within the University of Pennsylvania Medical System.

Inspired by the gift of a toy doctor's kit, Simon set himself on the physician's path early in life.

Simon was born to Jacqueline H. Simon and Joseph E. Simon in 1938 in Philadelphia. He graduated from Cheltenham High School in 1955 and Princeton University in 1959 with a Bachelor of Arts degree.

He then earned his medical degree in 1963 from the University of Pennsylvania Medical School. He completed his orthopedic training at Harvard University and returned to Philadelphia to practice medicine for the rest of his life.

During the Vietnam war, Simon served as a Lieutenant Commander and took care of soldiers at the Naval Hospital and Walter Reed. He also led numerous clinical research teams and published the results of that work at the National Institutes of Health Institute for Arthritis and metabolic diseases.

His love of music started early in childhood when he was a boy soprano. He continued to perform throughout his life with groups such as the Triangle Club at Princeton and The Good Time Charlies at Penn Medical School. Into his 80s he performed Cole Porter melodies with a group of retired friends.

He also penned a series of mystery novels with a medical twist that featured "a loveably quirky doctor as the main character that bore a striking resemblance to himself."

Manmohan Singh

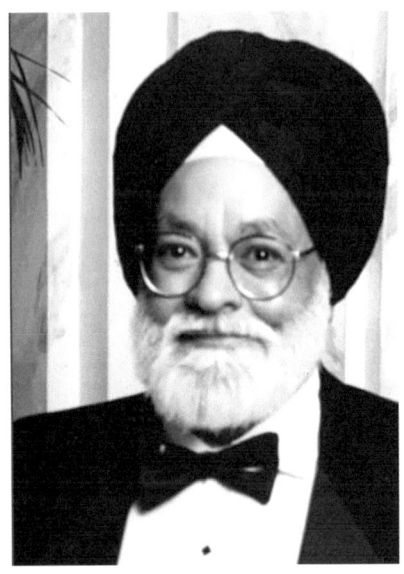

Born:	1939
Died:	2021
Years Active:	30+
Location:	Chicago, IL
Role(s):	Originator of the 'Singh Index'. Director of Orthopedic Research at Michael Reese Hospital

Manmohan Singh, M.D was the Director of Orthopedic Research at Michael Reese Hospital in Chicago, Illinois and the originator of the "Singh Index," a method used to predict the risk of hip fracture due to osteoporosis.

Singh was raised by his grandfather in Patiala, India. Although surrounded by love, he faced a lot of adversity early in life, including a childhood accident that left him with severe burns on his legs which caused an infection that almost killed him.

After medical school in India, Dr. Singh came to the U.S. on a Fulbright Scholarship in 1969 working with Drs. Mel Post and Leo Weinstein in the orthopedic department at Michael Reese Hospital in Chicago. Then after training at Mayo Clinic in Rochester, Minnesota, Singh became the director of orthopedic research at Michael Reese where he continued to explore better ways to diagnose and treat osteoporosis.

During his career, he also specialized in bone fracture, carpal tunnel syndrome, scoliosis, and sports medicine.

Robert Small

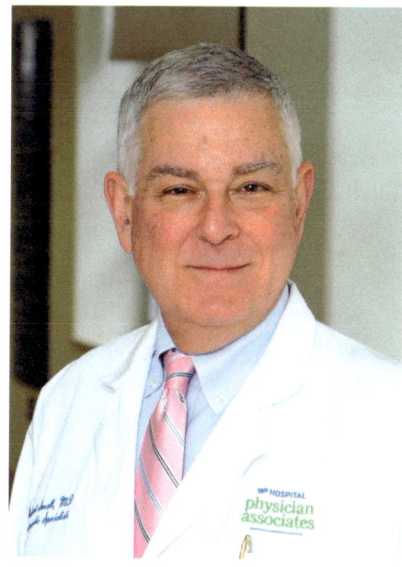

Dr. Robert Small was the Chief of the Orthopedic Institute and President of the Medical and Dental staff at White Plains, New York Hospital.

For more than 30 years, Dr. Small treated orthopedic patients in New York City and the White Plains region.

Hi undergraduate degree is from Tufts University and his medical degree was from New York Medical College, followed by an orthopedic residency at the Hospital for Joint Diseases, where he served as Chief Resident, and an orthopedic fellowship at the Hospital for Special Surgery in Manhattan.

Paul D. Fragner, M.D. of the Westchester Orthopaedic Institute said of Dr. Small, "My fondest memory of Bob Small is seeing him in the office, every day for 20 years, always in a good mood, happy to be there, and hearing his genuine concern and joyous laughter while talking with patients and their families."

Dot Berman, a nurse at White Plains Hospital, said of Dr. Small, "He was so talented as an orthopedic surgeon, and he loved the challenge of a difficult case. He could handle complicated joint revisions and complex fractures with great skill and often made it look easy. You could depend on him to come up with a solution if something unexpected happened intraoperatively. He was always so even tempered and pleasant…it was obvious he loved surgery!"

Born:	1952
Died:	2015
Years Active:	30+
Location:	New York
Role(s):	Chief of the Orthopedic Institute and President of the Medical and Dental Staff, White Plains Hospital. Chief resident and fellow at the Hospital for Special Surgery.

Otto K. Stewart

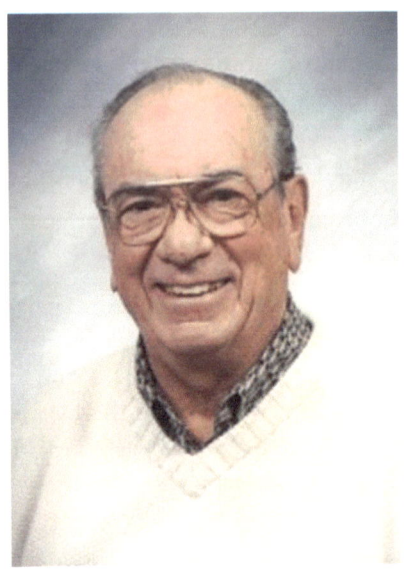

Otto K. Stewart, M.D., was president of St. Nicholas Hospital, chairman of the Piedmont Orthopedic Society, a member of the Sierra Cascade Trauma Society, a member of the American Academy of Orthopedic Surgeons, member, and a board member of the Bay Lakes Council of the Boy Scouts of America.

Otto Stewart was born in 1927 in Hornell, New York, to Otto K. and Lorene Driscoll Stewart. He attended Georgetown University for both undergraduate and medical school, finishing in 1952.

Dr. Stewart served in the U.S. Army Medical Reserve in Germany.

After his military service, Dr. Stewart completed his residency at Duke University where he was chief orthopedic resident.

After Duke University, Dr. Stewart and his wife relocated to Sheboygan, Wisconsin, where Dr. Stewart joined Dr. John Van Driest, his chief in Germany and started one of the first large joint arthroplasty practices in the area. The team were treated orthopedic patients at eight regional Wisconsin hospitals. Dr. Don Gore joined the partners in 1968.

Dr. James Urbaniak, spokesman for the Piedmont Orthopedic Society said of Dr. Stewart, "Dr. Otto Stewart finished his Duke Orthopaedic Residency in 1962. He and his wife Mickey faithfully attended the annual Piedmont Orthopaedic Society meetings for nearly 50 years. He was well known for the presentation of the Piedmont Kelley Award for the Scientific Session each year along with Glen Musselman. Otto and Glen also co-chaired the Piedmont Orthopedic Society annual meeting in 1981."

Born:	1927
Died:	2017
Years Active:	
Location:	Sheboygan, WI
Role(s):	President of the Piedmont Orthopedic Society, President of St. Nicholas Hospital and Pioneer orthopedic surgeon.

Elton Strauss

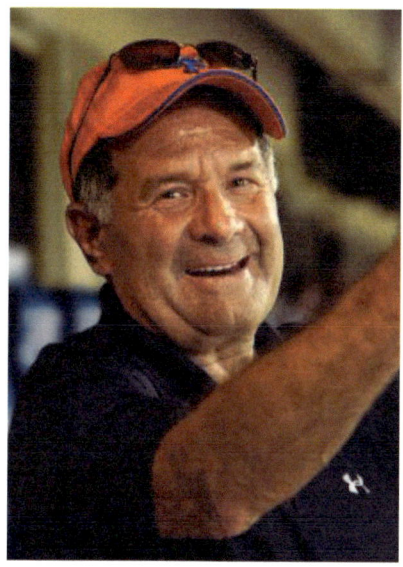

Born:	1948
Died:	2017
Years Active:	
Location:	New York City
Role(s):	Chief of Orthopaedic Trauma and Adult Reconstruction at Mount Sinai Hospital, Orthopedic surgery pioneer

Elton Strauss, M.D., was chief of Orthopaedic Trauma and Adult Reconstruction from 1984 to 2013 at The Mount Sinai Hospital in New York City.

Under Strauss, Sinai's resident clinic, usually the unacknowledged orphan of education, was transformed into a popular and outstanding component of the institution and made Sinai's residency program a model for a number of programs across the nation."

Born April 24, 1948, in Brooklyn, Elton Strauss earned his Bachelor of Science in biology from Long Island University C.W. Post in 1970, graduating from medical school at the University of Guadalajara in Mexico in 1974.

He completed his residency in orthopedic surgery at Bronx-Lebanon Hospital Center, Albert Einstein College of Medicine.

Dr. Strauss often saw nearly 100 patients on a Tuesday and Thursday, operate the rest of the week, and do follow-up rounds early Saturday morning.

Michael Hausman, M.D., Lippmann Professor of Orthopedic Surgery at Mount Sinai, added, "Elton has never, ever shirked from a challenge or a risk. He has always 'been there' for the house staff and for his patients. He has tackled unfashionable challenges, such as the orthopedic clinic, and made them work for the residents and patients alike."

Howard Sturtz

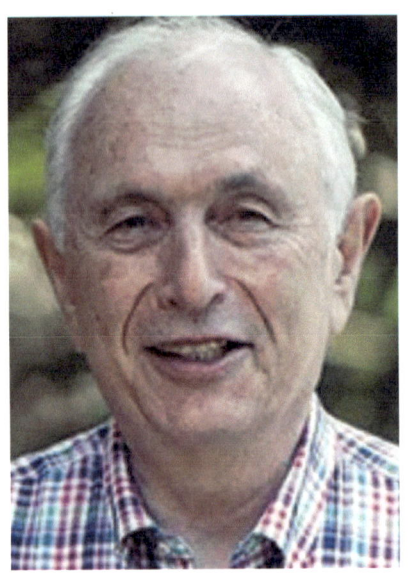

Born:	1935
Died:	2022
Years Active:	30+
Location:	Walnut Creek, CA
Role(s):	Pioneer orthopedic surgeon in the San Francisco Bay area

Howard Sturtz, M.D., earned his medical degree at the very moment large joint arthroplasty was being perfected in England and, in the Bay area, at both John Muir Medical Center and at Delta Memorial Hospital, Dr. Sturtz was an early advocate for many new orthopedic and surgical technologies.

At John Muir Medical Center, he was an arthroscopy pioneer, purchasing one of the first arthroscopic tools for that institution.

Dr. Sturtz was also part of the John Muir Trauma Team and Utilization Review Committee.

Later on in his career, he consulted with Bay Area orthopedic practices providing exams for the Social Security Administration, U.S. Department of Labor and expert reviews for the State Medical Board.

Sturtz was born on June 12, 1935, in Bronx, New York and spent his childhood there. As a teenager, he spent summers as a lifeguard at Rockaway Beach in Queens, New York. After high school, he attended Columbia University, graduating in 1956. He then received his medical degree from SUNY Downstate Medical School in Brooklyn in 1960.

Dr. Sturtz furthered his medical training with an orthopedic surgical residency at the Jewish Hospital in New York and a summer internship on a Native American reservation in Oklahoma in 1965.

Simultaneous with joining the staff of John Muir Medical Center, Dr. Sturtz established his own practice across the street from the hospital. He also had a practice in Antioch at Delta Memorial Hospital.

Dr. Sturtz was also president of the Contra Costa Chapter of American Friends of Magen David Adom and supported the people and the State of Israel with a gift of an ambulance.

Steven W. Theis

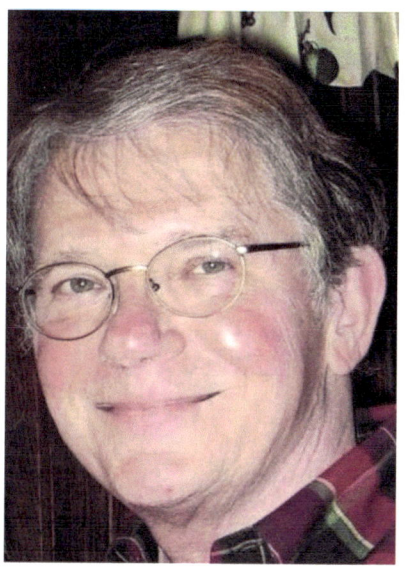

Born:	1943
Died:	2020
Years Active:	
Location:	Pittsburgh, PA
Role(s):	Chief of Orthopedic Surgery Elgin Air Force Base and Orthopedic Surgery pioneer in the Pittsburgh region

Steven W. Theis was the Chief of Orthopedic Surgery at Elgin Air Force Base, a Major in the United States Air Force and a early joint arthroplasty surgeon in the Pittsburgh area.

Born on September 24, 1943, in Barberton, Ohio, he spent much of his early years in Pennsylvania where he graduated from Mt. Lebanon High School. He then attended Wabash College in Crawfordsville, Indiana, and the graduated from the University of Pittsburgh School of Medicine.

After graduating medical school in 1969, Dr. Theis did his residency and a fellowship in orthopedic surgery at the University of Pittsburgh Medical Center, where he was chief resident.

Dr. Theis was also a major in the United States Air Force and Chief of Orthopedic Surgery at Elgin Air Force Base Regional Hospital. He was awarded the Air Force Commendation Medal in 1976.

Theis then went on to set up his own practice in Washington and Canonsburg, Pennsylvania, two suburbs just south of Pittsburgh. Before retiring in January 2013, he also spent several years with Advanced Orthopaedics and Rehab.

Michael Steven Thompson

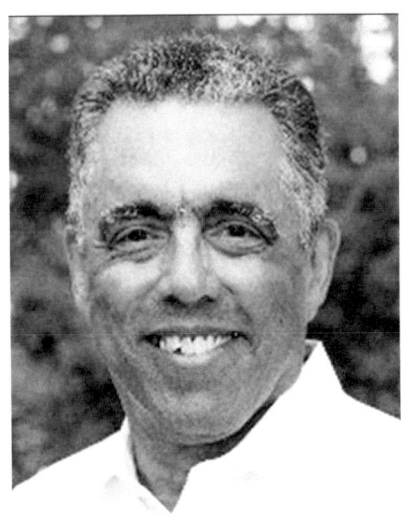

Michael Steven Thompson, M.D., became a surgeon and chose orthopedics at precisely the moment when joint arthroplasty was bursting on the scene.

Dr. Thompson was not only a pioneering arthroplasty surgeon, but he was a first adopter of such important new technologies as surgical training simulators.

Dr. Thompson came from a family of physicians and Ph.D. researchers. He completed his residency in 1977 at SUNY in Upstate New York and served the orthopedic needs of the Burlington, Massachusetts, community at both Lahey Hospital and Beverly Hospital, which are located in the north Boston suburbs, for nearly four decades.

Born:	1950
Died:	2022
Years Active:	38
Location:	Burlington, MA
Role(s):	Champion for early surgical simulation systems as educational tools for young orthopedic surgeons.

Dr. Thompson started his medical journey with a bachelor's degree of science from Columbia University in 1973. He quickly followed that with a medical degree from the State University of New York Upstate Medical University in Syracuse in 1977. His residency in general surgery was also at SUNY in Syracuse and then his orthopedic training came from Tufts New England Medical Center in Boston where he graduated in 1983.

Thompson's love for medicine and orthopedics started early when he and his brother Arthur played sports as kids. They ended up at the ER or the doctor's office many times throughout the years and it made an impression upon him.

Dr. Thompson was born on August 13, 1950, in New York City to his parents, Edna and Errol Thompson, M.D.

Thompson was an innovator whether he was in the operating room or at home. At Lahey Hospital, he was instrumental in establishing a surgical simulation center to train up and coming orthopedic surgeons.

Craig Tifford

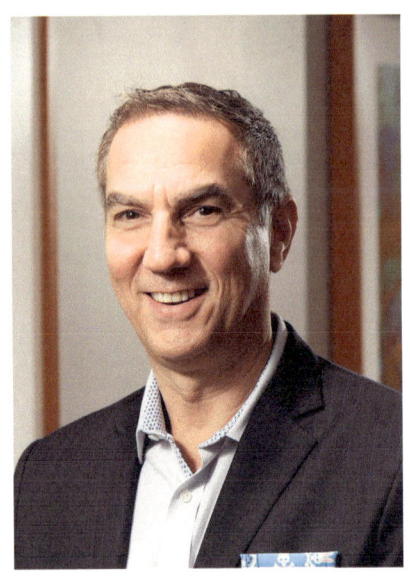

Born:	1968
Died:	2021
Years Active:	20+
Location:	Stamford, CT
Role(s):	Regional medical director Fairfield County for Yale Medicine and medical director of the Long Ridge Medical Center, prolific scientific and book chapter author

Orthopedic surgeon Craig Tifford, M.D. was regional medical director Fairfield County for Yale Medicine and medical director of the Long Ridge Medical Center in Stamford, Connecticut.

He was also an associate master instructor at the Orthopedic Learning Center in Rosemont, Illinois, where he helped teach arthroscopic surgery skills to surgeons from across the country and across the globe.

Dr. Tifford was board certified by the American Board of Orthopedic Surgery and sub-specialty board certified by the American Orthopedic Society for Sports Medicine. He was also a board member of the Connecticut Orthopaedic Society as well as actively involved with the American Academy of Orthopedic Surgery, the American Board of Orthopedic Surgery, and the Arthroscopy Association of North America.

Dr. Tifford was the author of many scientific papers and book chapters and presented and lectured at meetings across the country on athletic injuries, arthroscopy and reconstruction of the knee and shoulder joints.

Dr. Tifford was born on March 12, 1968, in Queens, New York to Lois Turner and Alan Tifford. He spent his childhood in Dix Hills, New York. His passion for music almost rivaled his passion for medicine. As a child, he played keyboard and then later in life picked up the drums. He was the drummer of a band Suburban Chaos that played gigs in the tri-state area.

He received his Bachelor of Science degree from Emory University in Atlanta and his medical degree from the Albert Einstein College of Medicine in Bronx, New York. He then went on to complete his orthopedic surgical residency at Montefiore Medical Center/Albert Einstein College of Medicine and a sports medicine fellowship at the Southern California Center for Sports Medicine in Long Beach, California.

Ralph Ilian Touma

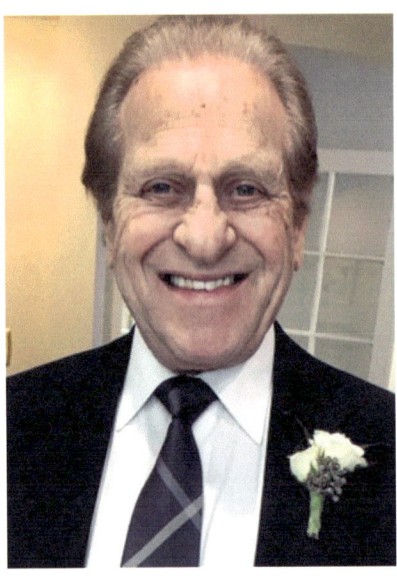

Born:	1942
Died:	2022
Years Active:	40+
Location:	Ashland, KY
Role(s):	Joint arthroplasty pioneer

Ralph Ilian Touma, M.D., was one of the first large joint arthroplasty surgeons to set up practice in the Ohio River town of Ashland, Kentucky and the surrounding rural Ohio and Kentucky region.

He served the area for more than four decades.

Dr. Touma was born in Damascus, Syria, to Ilian and Emilie Touma on December 16, 1942. He attended high school at the Lycée Francais and, later, medical school, at the University of Damascus in Damascus before moving to the United States in 1969 for his residencies.

He did his surgical residency at Pontiac General Hospital in Michigan and his orthopedic residency at the University of Illinois, Chicago.

From there, and this is, no doubt, an interesting story, he moved to the town of Ashland, Kentucky where he treated patients in his office and at Kings Daughters Medical Center also in Ashland.

"His love and respect for the art of medicine was understood by all who knew him…A man of great curiosity and intellect, he loved learning about history, listening to opera and classical music, and traveling the world," his family wrote.

He also was known as a very charitable man both with money and his time. He especially enjoyed volunteering at Shriner's Children's Hospital in Lexington.

Thomas Frank Trainer

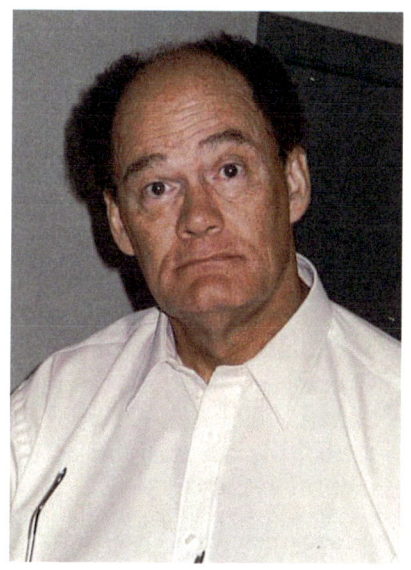

Born:	1940
Died:	2022
Years Active:	42
Location:	Indianapolis, IN
Role(s):	Chairman St. Vincent Department of Orthopedics, President of the Indiana Orthopedic Society

Dr. Thomas Frank Trainer was the chairman of St. Vincent's Department of Orthopedics in Indianapolis and past president of the Indiana Orthopedic Society.

Trainer's 42-year career encompassed virtually every phase in the development of modern orthopedics.

Dr. Trainer earned his medical degree from Indiana University in Bloomington in 1966. His internship was at Providence Hospital in Portland, Oregon, in 1967 and he was accepted into the residency program at West Virginia University Hospital in Morgantown, West Virginia, in 1968.

Trainer's career was spent primarily with the St. Vincent Hospital system—one of the larger national health systems with 143 hospitals and more than 40 senior living facilities in 19 states and the District of Columbia.

Dr. Trainer was awarded the most prestigious physician award by St. Vincent Hospitals. He also served as chairman of the St. Vincent Indianapolis Orthopedic Surgery Department for many years. Dr. Trainer was an active member of the Indiana Orthopedic Society and was, for a term, the society's president.

Dr. Trainer was born to Frank and Blanche Trainer in Evansville, Indiana in 1940. He grew up in Evansville, Indiana, where he attended Evansville Reitz High School. He played football there and also at Indiana University in Bloomington where he received his bachelor's and medical degrees.

Trainer was a member of The Lamb's Club, a professional theatric club first started in New York City, and the Player's Club, the oldest continuously operating community theatre organization in Marion County.

James Edwin White

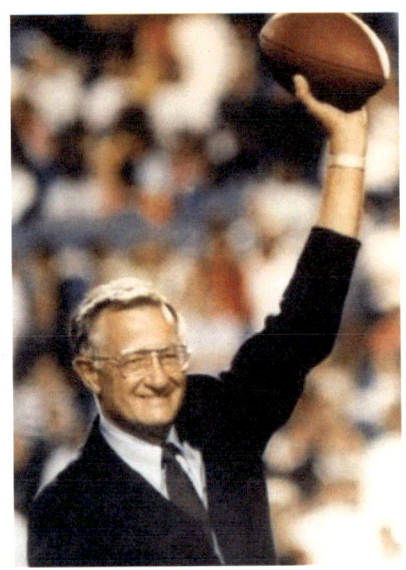

Born:	1929
Died:	2015
Years Active:	40+
Location:	Tulsa, Ok
Role(s):	Co-founder of Eastern Oklahoma Orthopedic center, Orthopedic and Sports Medicine Pioneer

James Edwin White, M.D., was co-founder of Eastern Oklahoma Orthopedic Center and a pioneer in Oklahoma sports medicine.

Dr. White was born in Okmulgee, Oklahoma and graduated from the University of Oklahoma medical school, completing his residency at the University of Minnesota. He then returned to Oklahoma, where he practiced in Tulsa, and in 1967 co-founded the Eastern Oklahoma Orthopedic Center with his partners John Smith and Jim Winslow.

George Mauerman, M.D. collaborated with his friend Dr. White for many years and said this about Dr. White, "I came to town in 1970 and at that point Jim was already covering high school sports. At that time, the American Orthopaedic Society for Sports Medicine (AOSSM) did not exist. Jim started covering the University of Tulsa athletic injuries and was instrumental in getting a number of other orthopedic surgeons interested in covering teams. We soon picked up a hockey team, a baseball team, a football team, and a local soccer team."

"You could not outwork him, in fact. He was very innovative with operative procedures that went on to be adopted by other orthopedic surgeons nationwide. One was the reconstruction of the ACL [anterior cruciate ligament] using the patellar tendon...and he adopted arthroscopy earlier that most orthopedic surgeons in Oklahoma."

"He built the Eastern Oklahoma orthopedic group from nothing to where we are today (12 surgeons and 3 Primary Care Sports Medicine Physicians). In 1990 he helped institute the first Residency Program for Primary Care Sports Medicine at our practice; we still have two that are trained per year."

Jeffrey Emel, M.D. said this about Dr. White, "I do nonsurgical orthopedics. Years ago, he said, 'We are sports surgeons, and we need a sports doctor too.' He was a visionary because at that time no one thought to care for the athlete in that way."

"Dr. White guided me during my residency; he taught me a lot of good techniques regarding physical exams, and he had an exceptional memory. He was always inquisitive and looked for ways to improve upon things."

Richard P. Whittaker

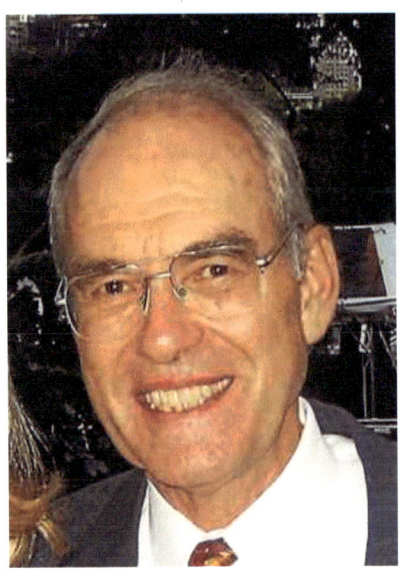

Born:	1941
Died:	2016
Years Active:	40+
Location:	Pottstown, PA
Role(s):	President of the Pennsylvania Medical Society, President Pennsylvania Orthopedic Society, Member of Pottstown Memorial Medical Center Board of Directors.

Richard P. Whittaker, M.D., was president of both Pennsylvania Medical Society and Pennsylvania Orthopedic Society and one of the original orthopedic surgeons in Montgomery County.

Dr. Whittaker received his medical degree from the University of Pennsylvania in 1966, at the very moment that orthopedics was being transformed from a fracture and bracing practice to a surgical one and completed a rotating internship and residency at Pennsylvania Hospital as well as a residency in orthopedic surgery at the Hospital of the University of Pennsylvania.

Dr. Whittaker served as a major in the U.S. Army Reserve and later moved to active-duty status, serving as a staff orthopedic surgeon from 1971 to 1974 in Panama.

He joined the Pottstown Memorial Medical Center staff in November 1974, and in 1977 was elected to the executive committee at the hospital. He served as a medical staff representative on the board of directors from 2003-2008 before becoming chairman of the board.

Richard Frantz is a member of the PMMC Board of Trustees said, of Dr. Whittaker, "During his 39-year tenure, Dr. Whittaker touched many lives by being a physician in the community he loved. Not only the lives of his patients, but also many of our nurses, physicians, and volunteers as well."

"People here fondly remember such stories about how he would cross-country ski into the ER during a snowstorm to personally check on his patients. Truly remarkable was his compassion and dedication to service."

"He volunteered his surgical skills all over the world including Panama, Guatemala, Nicaragua and most recently Haiti, where he served with Doctors Without Borders to aid the victims of the earthquake there."

"He proudly showed off his hip replacements and rode his bicycle 4,000 miles raising money for various charities. Near his 50th wedding anniversary, along with his family, friends, and his bride Peggy, rode 50 kilometers on the Schuylkill River Trail. And on his 70th birthday, he proudly rode seventy kilometers."

Robert Michael Yanchus

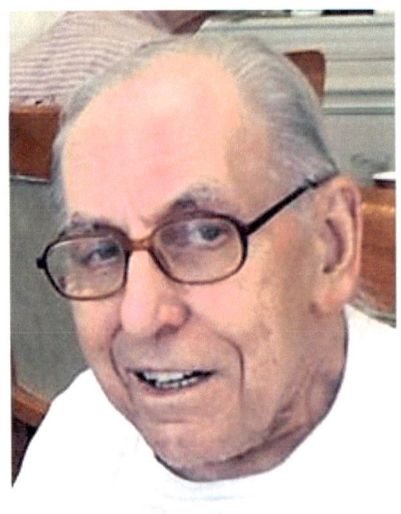

The Battle of the Bulge in 1945 turned 19-year old Robert Michael Yanchus into an orthopedic surgeon and earned him a Purple Heart.

For the majority of his career, Robert Michael Yanchus MD was an orthopedic surgeon at Citizens General Hospital in New Kensington and Allegheny Valley Hospital in Natrona Heights. He also had a private practice in New Kensington for many years.

It was that experience in World War II that changed Dr. Yanchus's life forever. Before that moment in the Ardennes forest, his goal in life had been to become a professional musician, a double bass player.

Yanchus was one of only three members of his platoon to survive the searing experience of the Battle of the Bulge and one of his good friends, a medic, died.

Yanchus came home dedicated to enter medicine. The GI bill paid his way through college and, eventually, prepared him for 50+ years of fixing broken bones and arthritic joints.

Born:	1926
Died:	2020
Years Active:	50+
Location:	Pittsburgh, PA
Role(s):	Pioneering Orthopedic Surgeon

Yanchus was the son of Czech and Hungarian immigrants and grew up in Masontown, Fayette County, just outside of Pittsburgh, graduating in 1943 from Masontown High School.

Dr. Yanchus earned a medical degree from the University of Pittsburgh School of Medicine in 1950 and chose orthopedic surgery as his specialty.

That was 9 years before John Charnley would give his famous lecture to a division of the British Medical Association, saying it was "probable" that a prosthetic "femoral prosthesis, articulating with a PTFE socket" would work.

Yanchus entered orthopedics just as the idea of hip arthroplasty was beginning to seem inevitable.

Yanchus's motivation for becoming an orthopedic surgeon was that it had a concrete patient outcome. From 1950 to 2000, Dr. Yanchus was among the first and, as it turned out, longest lasting fixer of broken bones, arthritic joints and more in Western Pennsylvania.

EPILOGUE

The orthopedists profiled in this book were part of a post-World War II forward-looking culture which transformed the practice of musculoskeletal medicine from bracing and fracture fixation to repair, reconstruction and regeneration.

The technological innovations they created were remarkable, but the truly breathtaking history is the personal one – which manifested one patient at a time, sitting at the bedside, explaining a new procedure, fixing mistakes (Charnley's 300 failed hip arthroplasties in a row before his Eureka moment, for example), trading lessons at seminars with colleagues, thousands of lab hours, puzzling out problems with engineers, working with the master communicators of orthopedics – the sales people – and relying on the organizers to keep this exploding medical practice from descending into entropy.

This was not their father's practice of medicine.

As we approach the 21st century's quarter year mark, musculoskeletal care is leaving the age of implants and instruments and entering the age of data.

There will never be another group quite like this Greatest Generation of Orthopedists.

Robin Young – 2023

ABOUT THE AUTHOR
Robin R. Young

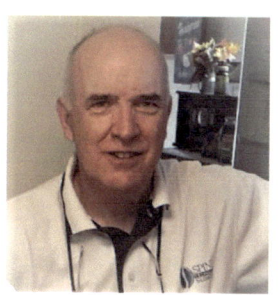

Robin Young is the founder and editor-in-chief of RRY Publications LLC, the publisher of Orthopedics This Week. He is also the founder of PearlDiver Technologies, Inc. a database company. Before starting his own publishing firm, Robin was an analyst and managing director for several Wall Street firms including Piper Jaffray, Stephens and HealthPoint Capital. For several years he was a member of the adjunct faculty for the Carlson School of Business at the University of Minnesota and the University of Saint Thomas. In the 1990s, he took a break from Wall Street to start a company named Clean Green Packing which invented the first starch based packing peanut. He has written thousands of articles, a handful of books, written, filed and received a patent for the use of amniotic fluid to treat knee arthritis and speaks at several medical meetings each year. He was born in Guatemala City, Guatemala and grew up in Cali, Columbia, Urbana, Illinois, Gallup, New Mexico and Canton, Ohio. Robin lives with his wife just outside of Portland, Oregon on the edge of the Willamette Valley and is usually in Sapporo, Japan for two to three months each year. He can be reached at robin@ryortho.com.

To be added:
John Insall
Rick Steedman